FRESH AND HEALTHY

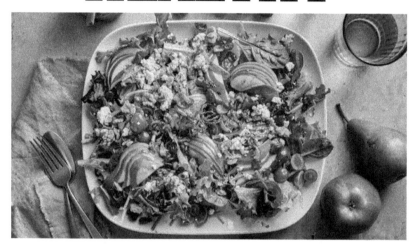

SALADS AND APPETIZERS

Gustav Mancini

Welcome!

..to this new series of book, inspired by all the recipes I know thanks to my great passion, **_cooking!_**

In this book you will find many different ideas for your dishes, with ingredients from all around the world, with a Gourmet touch!

Thanks to these cookbooks you can develop your cooking skills for any kind of meal,

as you'll find recipes for:

- Lunch
- Dinner
- Salads
- Desserts
- And much more...

Whether your favourite dish is French fries, muffins, chicken tenders or grilled vegetables, with this series of books you will learn how to do it with a better-looking touch!

If you think that it will be difficult to prepare a dish in a gourmet way, you will discover that it doesn't need that much to change the look of it.

Don't forget that this books have also low fat recipes with healthy ingredients to *keep you fit and have a healthier meal plan!*

Remember that having a wide variety of ingredients and foods in your diet have many benefits for you, that's why you will find ingredients from:

- Asia
- Russia
- America
- Europe
- And more...

Since I started to pay more attention on the decision of the ingredients and how to plate a dish, I enjoy cooking a lot more! That's why I made this cookbook for all of you that want to develop your cooking skills and start eating healthier!

I hope you will enjoy this book and don't forget to check out the other ones from the collection, and enjoy your time in the kitchen!

GOURMET RECIPES FOR BEGINNERS: SIDES

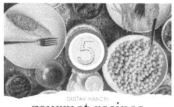

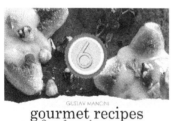

Learn how to cook delicious sides to enjoy your meals! This cookbook contains classy recipes to cook step-by-step, ideal to build a healthy and delicious meal plan, but also perfect for your events and parties!

GOURMET RECIPES FOR BEGINNERS: DESSERTS

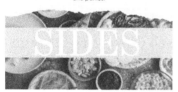

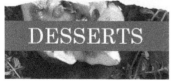

Learn how to cook quick desserts to give your day a good flavour! This cookbook contains easy but selected recipes to prepare step-by-step delicious desserts, snacks and pies, with fruit and other ingredients, Perfect for your events, parties and aperitifs or simply at the end of your dinner!

GOURMET RECIPES FOR BEGINNERS: SALADS

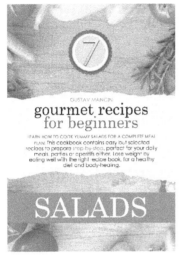

Learn how to cook yummy salads for a complete meal plan! This cookbook contains easy but selected recipes to prepare step-by-step, perfect for your daily meals, parties or aperitifs either. Lose weight by eating well with the right recipe book, for a healthy diet and body-healing.

GOURMET RECIPES FOR BEGINNERS: BREAD

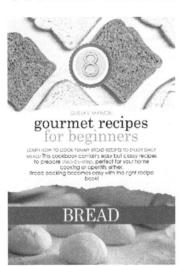

Learn how to cook yummy bread recipes to enjoy daily meals! This cookbook contains easy but classy recipes to prepare step-by-step, perfect for your home cooking or aperitifs either.
Bread backing becomes easy with the right recipe book!

GOURMET RECIPES FOR BEGINNERS: LUNCH

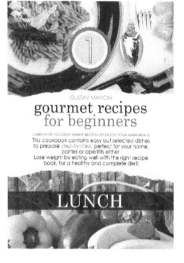

Learn how to cook yummy recipes to enjoy your main meals! This cookbook contains easy but selected dishes to prepare step-by-step, perfect for your home, parties or aperitifs either. Lose weight by eating well with the right recipe book, for a healthy and complete diet!

GOURMET RECIPES FOR BEGINNERS: DINNER

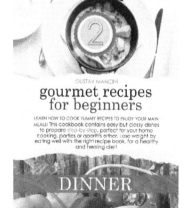

Learn how to cook yummy recipes to enjoy your main meals! This cookbook contains easy but classy dishes to prepare step-by-step, perfect for your home cooking, parties or aperitifs either. Lose weight by eating well with the right recipe book, for a healthy and healing diet!

GOURMET RECIPES FOR BEGINNERS:QUICK AND EASY

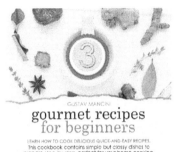

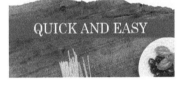

Learn how to cook delicious quick-and-easy recipes. This cookbook contains simple but classy dishes to prepare step-by-step, perfect for your home cooking, parties or aperitifs either. Lose weight by eating well with the right recipe book, for a healthy and TIME-SAVING diet!

GOURMET RECIPES FOR BEGINNERS: APPETIZERS

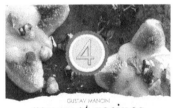

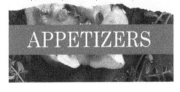

Learn how to cook tasty snacks to enjoy your free time! With many and different ingredients, this cookbook contains more than 50 appetizer recipes to cook step-by-step, ideal to build a healthy and delicious daily meal plan, but also perfect for your events, parties and aperitifs!!

FRESH AND HEALHTY SALADS AND APPETIZERS

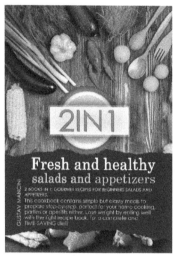

2 BOOKS IN **1**: gourmet recipes for beginners salads and appetizers. This cookbook contains simple but classy meals to prepare step-by-step, perfect for your home cooking, parties or aperitifs either. Lose weight by eating well with the right recipe book, for a complete and TIME-SAVING diet!

COMPLETE MEAL PLAN FOR BEGINNERS

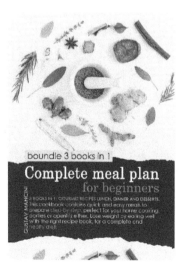

3 BOOKS IN **1**: gourmet recipes lunch, dinner and desserts. This cookbook contains quick and easy meals to prepare step-by-step, perfect for your home cooking, parties or aperitifs either. Lose weight by eating well with the right recipe book, for a complete and healthy diet!

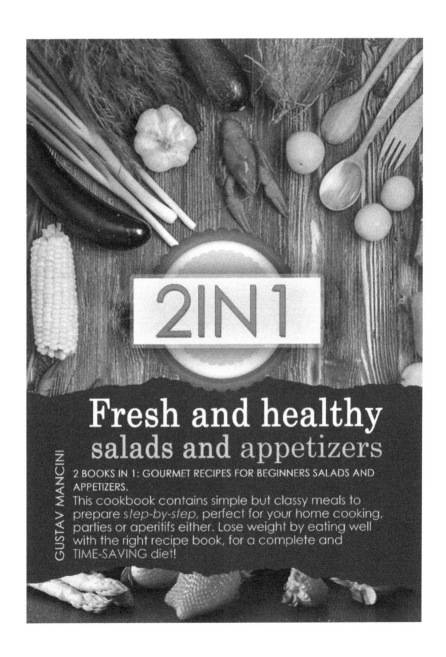

2IN1

Fresh and healthy
salads and appetizers

2 BOOKS IN 1: GOURMET RECIPES FOR BEGINNERS SALADS AND APPETIZERS.
This cookbook contains simple but classy meals to prepare *step-by-step*, perfect for your home cooking, parties or aperitifs either. Lose weight by eating well with the right recipe book, for a complete and TIME-SAVING diet!

GUSTAV MANCINI

Table of Contents

GOURMET RECIPES FOR BEGINNERS

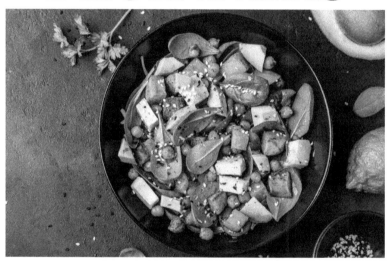

SALADS

SOME HEALTHY CHOICHES FOR YOUR MEAL

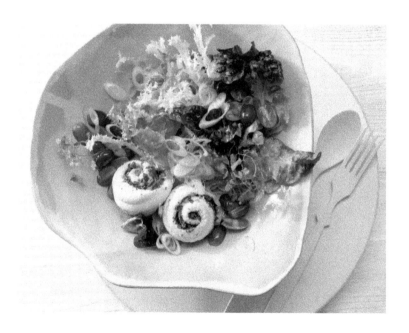

Asparagus And Pancetta Salad

Serving: 8

Ingredients

- 2 pounds asparagus, trimmed

- 4 tablespoons extra-virgin olive oil, divided

- 2 cloves garlic, minced

- 1/4 pound pancetta, cut crosswise into 1/8 inch sticks

- 3 tablespoons lemon juice

- 2 teaspoons Dijon mustard

Direction

- Fill a steamer with 1 inch of boiling water so that the asparagus is soaked in it. Let the asparagus cook for 2-6 minutes until it is soft yet still firm. Drain the cooked asparagus and place it in a bowl of ice water to let it cool down; place the cooled down cooked asparagus on paper towers to drain excess liquid then put it on the serving platter.

- Put 1 tablespoon of olive oil in a medium-sized saucepan placed on medium-low heat and let it heat up. Put in the garlic and sauté it in hot oil for 2-3 minutes until you can already smell the aroma. Put in the pancetta and keep cooking for 8-10 minutes while stirring until it turns brown in color.

- Move the pan away from heat and mix the lemon juice, Dijon and leftover 3 tablespoons of olive oil into the pancetta mixture. Drizzle the prepared sauce on top of the asparagus.

Nutrition Information

- Calories: 113 calories;
- Cholesterol: 5
- Protein: 4.3
- Total Fat: 8.8

- Sodium: 142

- Total Carbohydrate: 5.5

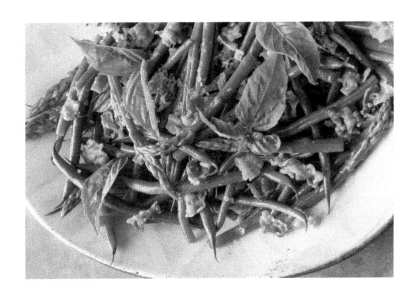

Antipasto Salad

Ingredients

- 8 ounces Genoa salami, cut into bite-size pieces

- 8 ounces sopressata or other hard salami, cut into bite-size pieces

- 8 ounces sharp provolone cheese, cut into bite-size pieces

- 8 ounces fresh mozzarella cheese, cut into bite-size pieces

- 2 large tomatoes, cut into bite-size pieces

- 1 (14 ounce) can artichokes, drained and cut into bite-size pieces

- 1/2 (12 ounce) jar roasted red peppers, drained and sliced

- 1/2 cup pitted and coarsely chopped Kalamata olives

- 1/4 cup pitted and chopped green olives

- 1 tablespoon extra-virgin olive oil

- 3 tablespoons red wine vinegar

- freshly-ground black pepper, to taste

- 1/4 cup shredded fresh basil leaves

Direction

Mix artichokes, tomatoes, mozzarella, provolone, sopressata salami and Genoa in a bowl. Slice roasted red peppers; add in the bowl with 3 tablespoons of the juice.

Mix chopped olives in; drizzle olive oil on the whole dish then black pepper and red wine vinegar. You can prepare salad ahead of time then refrigerate till serving.

Tear fresh basil leaves to bite-sized pieces; add to salad before serving. Mix well; serve.

Nutrition Information

- Calories: 383 calories;

- Sodium: 1783

- Total Carbohydrate: 7.9

- Cholesterol: 74

- Protein: 21.7

- Total Fat: 29.1

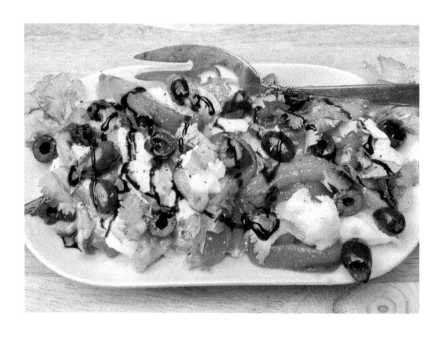

Apple, Avocado And Hearts Of Palm Salad

Serving: 6

Ingredients

1 cup mayonnaise

1/4 cup ketchup

1 tablespoon white sugar

1 lemon, juiced

1/4 teaspoon paprika

1 pinch ground black pepper

2 tablespoons chopped fresh chives

3 cups mixed salad greens

1 avocado - pitted, peeled, and cubed

2 Granny Smith apples - peeled, cored and sliced thin

1/2 cup coarsely chopped walnuts

1 cup sliced hearts of palm

Direction

Whisk pepper, paprika, lemon juice, sugar, ketchup and mayonnaise together in a small bowl. Add chives, stir well and set aside.

On individual serving plates, lay out the watercress. Place hearts of palm, avocado and apple on top. Add walnuts on top and sprinkle with dressing.

Drizzle the dressing evenly over salad and serve.

Nutrition Information

- Calories: 435 calories;
- Sodium: 434
- Total Carbohydrate: 19.5
- Cholesterol: 14
- Protein: 4.1
- Total Fat: 40.8

Apple Cranberry Salad

Serving: 4

Ingredients

1 teaspoon stone-ground mustard

2 tablespoons balsamic vinegar

1/4 cup olive oil

1 apple, diced

1 pear, diced

1/4 cup dried cranberries

1 (10 ounce) package mixed baby greens

1/4 cup crumbled blue cheese

2 tablespoons chopped walnuts

Direction

- In a small bowl, whisk together vinegar and mustard; while whisking, sprinkle in the olive oil to make a dressing; set aside.

- In a large salad bowl, put walnuts, blue cheese, baby greens, cranberries, pear and apple. Mix by tossing gently, pour dressing over salad, and toss until well coated.

Nutrition Information

- Calories: 256 calories;

- Total Fat: 18.6

- Sodium: 160

- Total Carbohydrate: 21.5

- Cholesterol: 6

- Protein: 3.7

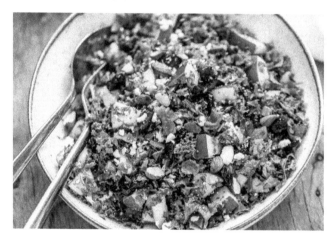

Arugula Persimmon Pear Salad

Ingredients

1 teaspoon Dijon mustard

1/2 lemon, juiced

1/4 cup olive oil

1 shallot, minced

1 persimmon, sliced

1 pear, sliced

1/2 cup walnut pieces, toasted

1 bunch arugula

1 tablespoon shaved Parmesan cheese

salt and pepper to taste

Direction

- Mix shallot, olive oil, lemon juice, and mustard in a bowl. Add arugula, walnuts, pear, and sliced persimmon and mix it well until coated.

- Top salad with shaved parmesan cheese and season with pepper and salt.

Nutrition Information

- Calories: 527 calories;

- Protein: 9.3

- Total Fat: 45.1

- Sodium: 140

- Total Carbohydrate: 30.7

- Cholesterol: 2

Arugula Salad With Citrus Vinaigrette

Serving: 4

Ingredients

- 1/3 cup freshly squeezed grapefruit juice

- 1/3 cup freshly squeezed orange juice

- 1/3 cup extra virgin olive oil

- salt to taste

- 6 ounces arugula - rinsed, dried and torn

- 1 pear, cored and sliced

- 1 red bell pepper, thinly sliced

Direction

- Mix salt, grapefruit juice, olive oil, and orange juice together in an airtight jar; shake well.

- Toss red pepper, pear, and arugula together in a salad bowl; pour in dressing. Mix well then serve.

Nutrition Information

- Calories: 229 calories;

- Sodium: 159

- Total Carbohydrate: 13.8

- Cholesterol: 0

- Protein: 1.8

- Total Fat: 19.1

Autumn Duck Confit Salad

Serving: 2

Ingredients

Salad:

2 cooked duck confit legs (with thighs attached)

1 cup curly endive (frisee)

1 cup arugula

1 cup chopped radicchio

1/2 cup purple grapes

1/2 cup peeled and minced apple

1/4 cup thinly sliced white turnip

1/4 cup coarsely chopped pecans

Dressing:

3 tablespoons olive oil

1 tablespoon maple syrup

1 tablespoon red wine vinegar

salt and ground black pepper to taste

Direction

- Preheat the oven to 350°F (175°C) Put the duck on a baking tray.

- Cook in the oven for 7 minutes, until heated through.

- Combine arugula, curly endive, grapes, turnip, apple, radicchio, and pecans in a big bowl.

- Toss in maple syrup, salt, pepper, olive oil, and vinegar in a bowl. Whisk it and pour over the salad. Mix well to coat every ingredient.

- Divide the salad into two bowls. Top salad with duck confit.

Nutrition Information

- Calories: 425 calories;

- Total Fat: 33.9

- Sodium: 138

- Total Carbohydrate: 23.6

- Cholesterol: 33

- Protein: 10.5

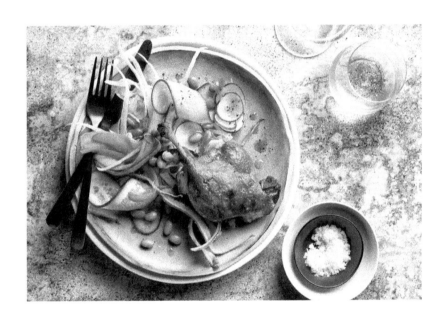

Balsamic Vinegar Potato Salad

Serving: 8

Ingredients

- 10 medium red potatoes, diced

- 1 small onion, chopped

- 1/2 cup diced roasted red peppers

- 1 (4 ounce) can sliced black olives, drained

- 1 (10 ounce) can quartered artichoke hearts, drained

- 1/2 cup balsamic vinegar

- 3 teaspoons olive oil

- 1 teaspoon dried oregano

- 1 teaspoon dried basil

- 1/2 teaspoon mustard powder

- 2 tablespoons chopped fresh parsley

Direction

- Cover potatoes with enough water in a saucepan. Boil then cook till tender, for 5-10 minutes. Let drain and move to a large bowl.

- Add artichokes, olives, red peppers and onion to the potatoes bowl. Whisk together parsley, mustard powder, basil, oregano, olive oil and balsamic vinegar in a separate bowl. Spread over the vegetables and stir till coated. Before serving, let chill for at least 4 hours to overnight.

Nutrition Information

- Calories: 257 calories;

- Total Fat: 3.9

- Sodium: 407

- Total Carbohydrate: 51.1

- Cholesterol: 0

- Protein: 6.9

Beet Salad With Goat Cheese

Serving: 6

Ingredients

- 4 medium beets - scrubbed, trimmed and cut in half

- 1/3 cup chopped walnuts

- 3 tablespoons maple syrup

- 1 (10 ounce) package mixed baby salad greens

- 1/2 cup frozen orange juice concentrate

- 1/4 cup balsamic vinegar

- 1/2 cup extra-virgin olive oil

- 2 ounces goat cheese

Direction

- Cover beets with enough water in saucepan; boil. Cook till tender for 20-30 minutes. Drain; cool. Cut to cubes.

- Put walnuts in skillet on medium low heat as beets cook; heat till beginning to toast and warm; mix maple syrup in. Mix and cook till coated evenly; take off heat. Put aside; cool.

- Whisk olive oil, balsamic vinegar and orange juice concentrate in small bowl for dressing.

- On each of 4 salad plates, put big helping of baby greens; evenly divide candied walnuts then sprinkle on greens. Put even amount of beets on greens; put dabs of goat cheese on top. Drizzle some dressing on each plate.

Nutrition Information

- Calories: 347 calories;
- Protein: 5.3
- Total Fat: 26.1
- Sodium: 107

- Total Carbohydrate: 25

- Cholesterol: 7

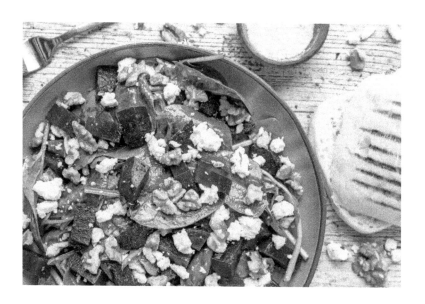

Bocconcini Salad

Serving: 4

Ingredients

1 pound bocconcini (bite-size mozzarella balls)

8 cherry tomatoes, halved

1/2 cup chopped green bell pepper

1/2 cup chopped celery

1/2 cup Belgian endive leaves

1/2 cup coarsely chopped arugula, stems included

1 1/2 tablespoons fresh lemon juice

3 tablespoons extra virgin olive oil

2 tablespoons chopped fresh basil leaves

salt and freshly ground black pepper

Direction

Combine arugula, endive, celery, bell pepper, cherry tomatoes and mozzarella in a large salad bowl.

Add olive oil and lemon juice together, whisk properly then pour over the salad. Toss well in order that all ingredients are well coated with dressing. Move salad to individual serving plates if needed. Sprinkle basil on top of salad; add salt and pepper to season, serve immediately.

Nutrition Information

- Calories: 448 calories;
- Total Fat: 35.7
- Sodium: 875
- Total Carbohydrate: 6.2
- Cholesterol: 90
- Protein: 25.9

Bulgur Chickpea Salad

Serving: 7

Ingredients

- 1 cup bulgur

- 2 cups boiling water

- 1/2 cup vegetable oil

- 1/2 cup fresh lemon juice

- salt to taste

- ground black pepper to taste

- 1 cup chopped green onions

- 1 (15 ounce) can garbanzo beans, drained

- 1 cup chopped fresh parsley

- 1 cup grated carrots

Direction

- Prepare a heatproof bowl, add in bulgur, and pour boiling water over bulgur. Allow to stand for 1 hour at room temperature.

- Beat together pepper, salt, lemon juice, and oil in a small bowl. Pour the mixture over bulgur, use a fork to mix properly.

- In a nice glass serving bowl, place bulgur in the bottom. On top of the bulgur, place layers of garbanzo beans and vegetables in this order: green onions, garbanzo beans, parsley, and carrots on top. Cover the bowl, put in the refrigerator to keep cold. Toss well just before serving

Nutrition Information

Calories: 273 calories;

Protein: 5.2

Total Fat: 16.6

California Cherry And Walnut Salad

Serving: 4

Ingredients

- 1 (10 ounce) bag mixed salad greens

- 1/4 cup raspberry vinaigrette

- 1/4 cup walnut pieces

- 2 tablespoons dried tart cherries

- 4 ounces goat cheese, sliced

- 1/4 pound cooked chicken breast strips

Direction

- In a large bowl, add dried cherries, walnut pieces, raspberry vinaigrette and salad greens, toss until well mixed.

- Distribute salad into individual salad plates or bowls.

- Decorate each salad with few chicken breast strips and two slices of goat cheese.

Nutrition Information

- Calories: 254 calories;

- Sodium: 401

- Total Carbohydrate: 13.4

- Cholesterol: 44

- Protein: 16.5

- Total Fat: 15.6

Caprese Salad With Balsamic Reduction

Serving: 4

Ingredients

- 1 cup balsamic vinegar

- 1/4 cup honey

- 3 large tomatoes, cut into 1/2-inch slices

- 1 (16 ounce) package fresh mozzarella cheese, cut into 1/4-inch slices

- 1/4 teaspoon salt

- 1/4 teaspoon ground black pepper

- 1/2 cup fresh basil leaves

- 1/4 cup extra-virgin olive oil

Direction

- In a small saucepan, stir together honey and balsamic vinegar, place saucepan over high heat. Bring mixture to a boil, lower the heat to low and simmer for about 10 minutes or until the amount of vinegar mixture decreases to 1/3 cup. Set aside the balsamic reduction and allow it to cool.

- On a serving platter, lay out mozzarella cheese and slices of tomatoes decoratively. Add salt and black pepper to season, put fresh basil leaves on top of the salad, and drizzle salad with balsamic reduction and olive oil.

Nutrition Information

Calories: 580 calories;

Total Fat: 38.8

Sodium: 331

Total Carbohydrate: 34.8

Cholesterol: 89

Protein: 22

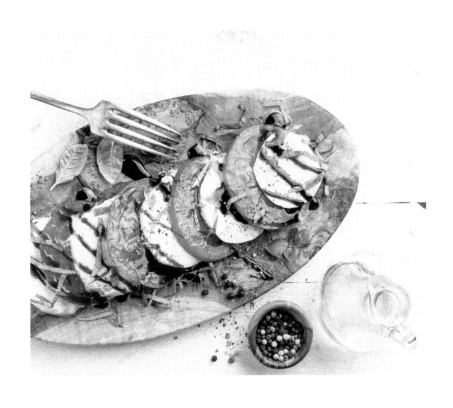

Cashew Curry Spinach Salad

Serving: 6

Ingredients

- Dressing:

- 1/2 cup vegetable oil

- 3 tablespoons red wine vinegar

- 3 tablespoons Dijon mustard

- 3 tablespoons sesame seeds

- 2 tablespoons honey

- 1 teaspoon chopped garlic

- Salad:

- 1/2 pound bacon

- 12 cups spinach leaves

- 6 cups coarsely chopped frisee (French curly endive)

- 3 small pears, thinly sliced

- 2/3 red onion, thinly sliced

- 6 grapes, halved (optional)

- Cashews:

- 3/4 cup raw cashews

- 1 tablespoon butter

- 1 tablespoon brown sugar

- 1 teaspoon curry powder

- 1 teaspoon dried rosemary

- 1/2 teaspoon salt

- 1/8 teaspoon cayenne pepper

Direction

- To make dressing, mix together garlic, honey, sesame seeds, Dijon mustard, red wine vinegar and vegetable oil in a bowl.

- In a large skillet, place in bacon and cook over medium-high heat, flip occasionally for about 10 minutes until turn brown evenly. Put bacon slices on paper towel to drain. Crumble into small pieces.

- On an individual serving plates, layer bacon crumbles, spinach leaves, frisee, pears, red onion, and grapes.

- Set oven to 400°F (200°C) and start preheating. Spread cashews evenly on a baking sheet.

- In a saucepan, melt butter over low heat. Add in cayenne pepper, salt, rosemary, curry powder and brown sugar, stir well until the mixture is smooth.

- In the preheated oven, toast cashew for 8 to 10 minutes until turn lightly brown. Add in cashew to the saucepan with butter mixture; stir until well coated. Allow to cool for about 10 minutes. Add cashew in salad plates, drizzle dressing over and serve

Nutrition Information

Calories: 481 calories;

Total Fat: 35.7

Sodium: 746

Total Carbohydrate: 33.9

Cholesterol: 19

Protein: 11.5

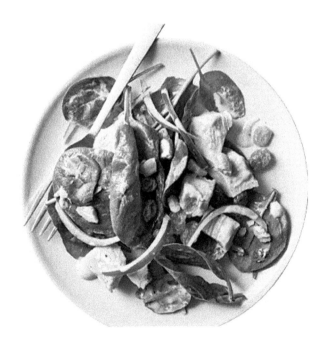

Cherry Chicken Salad

Serving: 4

Ingredients

3 cooked, boneless chicken breast halves, diced

1/3 cup dried cherries

1/3 cup diced celery

1/3 cup toasted, chopped pecans

1/3 cup low-fat mayonnaise

1 tablespoon buttermilk

1/2 teaspoon salt

1/2 teaspoon ground black pepper

1/3 cup cubed apples (optional)

Direction

- Mix chicken, pepper, dried cherries, salt, celery, milk, nuts, and mayonnaise together in a big bowl.

- Apple can be added as well if desired.

- Combine together and place in the refrigerator until cold.

- Serve salad with croissants or toasted cracked wheat bread.

Nutrition Information

- Calories: 264 calories;

- Sodium: 356

- Total Carbohydrate: 12

- Cholesterol: 62

- Protein: 24.3

- Total Fat: 12.7

Chicken Salad With Couscous

Serving: 6

Ingredients

- 1 cup couscous

- 2 cups chicken broth

- 1/2 cup dry white wine

- 2 teaspoons olive oil

- 2 tablespoons fresh lime juice

- 1 1/2 teaspoons ground cumin

- 1 clove garlic, minced

- 1 pound skinless, boneless chicken breast meat - cubed

- 1 green bell pepper, cut into large chunks

- 1 red bell pepper, cut into large chunks

- 1 yellow bell pepper, cut into large chunks

- 4 green onions, chopped
- 1/4 cup pitted black olives

Direction

Prepare couscous pasta based on package directions, use chicken broth for the liquid. Drain off and set aside.

Combine garlic, 1 teaspoon cumin, 1 tablespoon lime juice, oil and wine in a large skillet, mix well, and put in chicken. Set the heat to low to simmer for 5 to 7 minutes or until chicken juices run clear and all liquid fully evaporates.

Move chicken from the skillet to a large bowl, add couscous, green onion, yellow bell pepper, red bell pepper, green bell pepper, leftover 1 tablespoon lime juice and remaining 1/2 teaspoon cumin, mix well. Decorate per serving with few black olives.

Nutrition Information

- Calories: 281 calories;
- Protein: 25.9
- Total Fat: 4.5
- Sodium: 633

- Total Carbohydrate: 29.5

- Cholesterol: 45

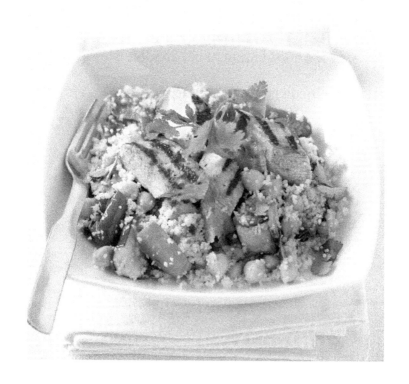

Conch Salad

Serving: 8

Ingredients

- 1 pound fresh conch

- 1 1/4 cups lemon juice, divided

- 1 cup diced tomatoes

- 1/2 cup diced onion

- 1/2 cup diced green bell pepper

- 1/2 cup diced cucumber

- 1/4 teaspoon seasoning blend (such as Badia® Complete Seasoning®), or to taste

- 1 pinch seasoned salt, or to taste

- 2 cups tomato juice

- 1/4 cup lime juice

- 1/4 cup vinegar

- 1 dash hot sauce, or to taste

Direction

Use meat mallet to tenderized conch. Cut into bite-size pieces. Prepare 1 cup of lemon juice, add in conch to soak for at least 2 hours, better if soak overnight.

Remove conch from lemon juice and place in a bowl. Add in seasoned salt, seasoning blend, cucumber, green pepper, onion and tomatoes, mix well.

Move conch mixture to a container. Add in lime juice, tomato juice and remaining of 1/4 cup lemon juice, mix properly. Add in hot sauce and vinegar, stir well. Put in the refrigerator and keep cold for about 1 hour until the flavors are well combined. Serve cold

Nutrition Information

- Calories: 111 calories;

- Protein: 14.6

- Sodium: 320

- Total Carbohydrate: 13.5

- Cholesterol: 37

- Total Fat: 0.3

Couscous Feta Salad

Ingredients

- 2 cups water

- 1 1/3 cups couscous

- 1 teaspoon salt

- 1/2 teaspoon ground black pepper

- 2 tablespoons red wine vinegar

- 1 1/2 tablespoons Dijon mustard

- 1/2 cup olive oil

- 1 cucumber, seeded and chopped

- 1 (4 ounce) container crumbled feta cheese

- 6 green onions, chopped

- 1/2 cup chopped fresh parsley

- 1/4 cup toasted pine nuts

Direction

Boil water in a saucepan over high heat. Remove it from the heat. Mix in couscous. Cover the pan and allow it to stand for 10 minutes. Scrape the couscous into the mixing bowl. Use a fork to fluff the couscous. Refrigerate it for 1 hour until cold.

Make the dressing once the couscous is cold by mixing the red wine vinegar, Dijon mustard, salt, and black pepper in a small bowl. Drizzle in olive oil slowly while mixing the mixture until the oil has thickened the dressing. Fold in feta cheese, pine nuts, parsley, cucumber, and green onions into the couscous. Pour the dressing all over the top and mix until evenly moistened. Before serving, let the mixture chill first for 30 minutes.

Nutrition Information

- Calories: 304 calories;
- Total Fat: 18.9
- Sodium: 528
- Total Carbohydrate: 26.8
- Cholesterol: 13

Cranberry Pecan Salad

Serving: 6

Ingredients

- 1 cup pecan halves

- 2 tablespoons raspberry vinegar

- 1/2 teaspoon Dijon mustard

- 1/2 teaspoon sugar

- 1/2 teaspoon salt

- freshly ground black pepper to taste (optional)

- 6 tablespoons olive oil

- 6 cups mixed salad greens, rinsed and dried

- 3/4 cup dried cranberries

- 1/2 medium red onion, thinly sliced

- crumbled feta cheese

Direction

- Set oven at 400°F (200°C) and start preheating. On a baking sheet, spread pecans evenly.

- Put pecans in the oven and toast for 8 to 10 minutes or until turn lightly brown and scented.

- Stir salt, pepper, sugar, mustard and vinegar together in a small bowl; mix well until salt and sugar dissolve fully in the liquid. Add in olive oil, whisk properly.

- Toss cheese, onions, pecans, cranberries and the greens together in a salad bowl. Pour in vinaigrette, toss lightly to coat salad with vinaigrette.

Nutrition Information

- Calories: 456 calories;
- Total Fat: 38.6
- Sodium: 780
- Total Carbohydrate: 21

- Cholesterol: 45

- Protein: 10

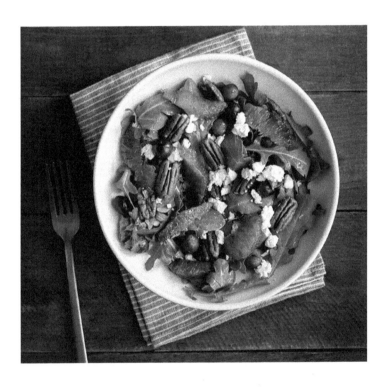

Cucumber Mango Salad With Citrus Vinaigrette

Serving: 4

Ingredients

- 1 English cucumber

- 1 mango

- 1 orange, juiced

- lemon, juiced

- 3 tablespoons grapefruit vinegar

- 4 leaves basil

- 1 pinch kosher salt

- 1 pinch ground black pepper

- 1/4 cup extra-virgin olive oil

Direction

- Remove cucumber skin. Use the vegetable peeler to peel strips of cucumber until you reach the soft core on all sides. Throw away cucumber core and skin. Put cucumber strips in a bowl.

- Remove mango skin. Use the vegetable peeler to peel strips of mango until you reach the seed on all sides. Throw away mango seed and skin. Put mango strips in the same bowl with cucumber.

- In a blender, combine black pepper, salt, basil, vinegar, lemon juice and orange juice, and puree. Slowly add in oil while blender is running. Pour dressing over cucumber and mango, mix well. Cover the bowl and keep cold for at least 2 hours

Nutrition Information

- Calories: 188 calories;

- Total Fat: 14.3

- Sodium: 103

- Total Carbohydrate: 17.2

- Cholesterol: 0

- Protein: 1.3

Dandelion Salad

Serving: 4

Ingredients

- 1/2 pound torn dandelion greens

- 1/2 red onion, chopped

- 2 tomatoes, chopped

- 1/2 teaspoon dried basil

- salt and pepper to taste

Direction

- Toss together tomatoes, red onion and dandelion greens in a medium bowl.

- Add salt, pepper and basil to taste.

Nutrition Information

- Calories: 42 calories;

- Sodium: 192

- Total Carbohydrate: 9

- Cholesterol: 0

- Protein: 2.3

- Total Fat: 0.5

Denise Salad Number One

Serving: 6

Ingredients

- 2 bunches arugula - rinsed, dried and torn

- 2 (11 ounce) cans mandarin orange segments, drained

- 1 large red onion, thinly sliced

- 1 pint cherry tomatoes

- 2 yellow bell peppers, seeded and diced

- 1 cup unsalted sunflower seeds

- 1/4 pound crumbled goat cheese

- 2 avocados - peeled, pitted and sliced

Direction

- Combine yellow peppers, tomatoes, onion, oranges and arugula in a large bowl.

- Choose your favorite dressing and add in the mixture.

- Add avocados, goat cheese and sunflower seeds on top then serve.

Nutrition Information

- Calories: 266 calories;

- Sodium: 136

- Total Carbohydrate: 26.2

- Cholesterol: 15

- Protein: 9.3

- Total Fat: 16.3

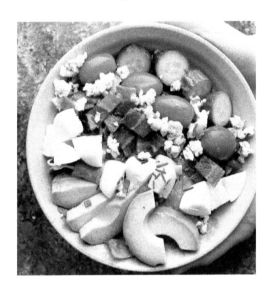

Detox Salad

Serving: 2

Ingredients

- 1 tablespoon cottage cheese

- 1 clove garlic, minced

- 1 teaspoon cider vinegar

- 1 tablespoon walnut oil

- salt and pepper to taste

- 2 Belgian endives, trimmed and leaves separated

- 1 apple, thinly sliced

- 1/2 cup stemmed watercress leaves

- 1/2 cup chopped walnuts

- 1/4 cup crumbled blue cheese

Direction

- In a small mixing bowl, mash together garlic and cottage cheese with a fork until smooth. Put in salt, pepper, walnut oil and cider vinegar, mix until well blended. Set aside.

- On two plates, lay out Belgian endive leaves in a circle as the tips point out. In the center of the plates, place apple, sprinkle with blue cheese, walnuts and watercress. Pour cottage cheese dressing over salads and serve.

Nutrition Information

- Calories: 370 calories;

- Total Fat: 30.9

- Sodium: 267

- Total Carbohydrate: 18.6

- Cholesterol: 13

- Protein: 9.9

Easy Arugula Salad

Serving: 4

Ingredients

- 4 cups young arugula leaves, rinsed and dried
- 1 cup cherry tomatoes, halved
- 1/4 cup pine nuts
- 2 tablespoons grapeseed oil or olive oil
- 1 tablespoon rice vinegar
- salt to taste
- freshly ground black pepper to taste
- 1/4 cup grated Parmesan cheese
- 1 large avocado - peeled, pitted and sliced

Direction

- Prepare a large plastic bowl that comes with a lid. In the bowl, combine Parmesan cheese, vinegar, oil, pine nuts, cherry tomatoes and arugula. Add salt and pepper to taste. Put the lid on to cover and shake until ingredients are well mixed.

- Separate salad onto plates, put avocado slices on top and serve

Nutrition Information

- Calories: 257 calories;

- Total Fat: 23.2

- Sodium: 381

- Total Carbohydrate: 10

- Cholesterol: 4

- Protein: 6.2

Eggplant Salad With Feta And Pomegranate

Serving: 4

Ingredients

2 eggplants, sliced

1 tablespoon salt, divided

1 cup yogurt

1 lemon, juiced

2 tablespoons olive oil

1 teaspoon ground black pepper

2 tomatoes, chopped

1 cucumber, chopped

1 pomegranate, seeds only

1/4 cup feta cheese

Direction

- Set an outdoor grill to medium heat and start preheating, lightly glaze the grate with oil. Sprinkle eggplant slices with 1/2 tablespoon salt to season.

- Cook eggplant on preheated oven for 10 to 15 minutes or until it becomes soft, remember to flip halfway through. Move to a platter and layout eggplant in a single layer.

- In a bowl, put black pepper, remaining 1/2 tablespoon salt, olive oil, lemon juice and yogurt, whisk well.

- Pour yogurt dressing on top of eggplant. Add cucumber and tomatoes on top. Sprinkle on top with feta cheese and pomegranate seeds.

Nutrition Information

- Calories: 284 calories;

- Total Carbohydrate: 41.5

- Cholesterol: 18

- Protein: 10.4

Elegant Brunch Chicken Salad

Ingredients

- 1 pound skinless, boneless chicken breast halves

- 1 egg

- 1/4 teaspoon dry mustard

- 1/2 teaspoon salt

- 2 teaspoons hot water

- 1 tablespoon white wine vinegar

- 1 cup olive oil

- 2 cups halved seedless red grapes

- 1 cup coarsely chopped pecans

- 1 cup coarsely crumbled blue cheese

Direction

- In a large pot, put in water and bring to a boil. Add in chicken and simmer for approximately 10 minutes until cooked well. Drain the chicken, let it cool and cut into cubes

- When chicken is boiling, make mayonnaise: Prepare a hand-held electric mixer or blender, use it to beat vinegar, water, salt, mustard and egg together until frothy and light. Add in one tablespoon of oil at a time, after each tablespoon of oil, beat thoroughly. When mixture starts to thickened, you can add oil more frequently. Continue to beat until mixture achieves the consistent and creamy texture of a mayonnaise.

- NOTE: The thickness of mayonnaise depends on the amount of oil you put in, it will get thicker if you add more oil; the full cup of oil might not be necessary

- Mix together 1 cup of homemade mayonnaise, blue cheese, pecans, grapes and chicken in a large bowl. Stir until salad is coated evenly, add more mayonnaise if needed. Keep cold until serving

Nutrition Information

Calories: 657 calories;

Total Carbohydrate: 12.6

Cholesterol: 92

Protein: 25.4

Total Fat: 57.7

Sodium: 571

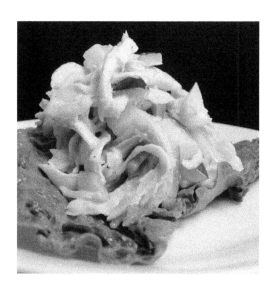

Roasted Vegetable Salad

Serving: 10

Ingredients

- 1 eggplant - quartered lengthwise, and sliced into 1/2 inch pieces

- 2 small yellow squash, halved lengthwise and sliced

- 4 cloves garlic, peeled

- 1/4 cup olive oil, or as needed

- 1 red bell pepper, seeded and sliced into strips

- 1 bunch fresh asparagus, trimmed and cut into 2 inch pieces

- 1/2 red onion, sliced

- 1/4 cup red wine vinegar

- 2 tablespoons balsamic vinegar

- 1/4 cup olive oil

- 2 lemons, juiced

- 1/4 cup chopped fresh parsley

- 3 tablespoons chopped fresh oregano

- salt and freshly ground black pepper to taste

Direction

Set an oven to 450°C (230°F). Grease a large baking sheet.

On the prepared baking sheet, evenly lay out eggplant and quash slices in layer. Place garlic cloves in one side of the pan so they can be found easily later. Bake in the preheated oven for 15 minutes.

While roasting the vegetables, put lemon juice, olive oil, balsamic vinegar and red wine vinegar together in a large serving bowl, whisk until well combined. Add salt, pepper, parsley and oregano to season. Remove cloves of garlic from the oven and mash or chop into smaller pieces. Add garlic to dressing, whisk well and set aside.

Remove vegetables from the oven, and stir the eggplant and the squash well. Place asparagus, red onion and red bell pepper in layer on top of squash and eggplant. Put back in the oven and bake for an additional 15 to 20 minutes or until asparagus becomes soft but still has bright green color.

Remove them from oven once vegetables are cooked well and slightly toasted. Place them in a bowl, pour in dressing, and stir until evenly coated. Taste and adjust the amount of salt and pepper if needed. Allow to chill for a few hours to marinate the vegetables.

Nutrition Information

Calories: 139 calories;

Total Carbohydrate: 10.8

Cholesterol: 0

Protein: 2.4

Total Fat: 11.2

Sodium: 64

Ensalada De Nopales (Mexican Cactus Salad)

Serving: 4

Ingredients

2 nopales (cactus pads)

3 tablespoons olive oil, divided

salt and ground black pepper to taste

4 Roma tomatoes, thinly sliced

2 serrano chiles, thinly sliced

1/2 cup thinly sliced pickled red onion, or to taste

1 lime, juiced

2 tablespoons finely chopped cilantro

1 teaspoon dried oregano

2 tablespoons cotija cheese

2 avocados, halved and pitted

2 tablespoons roasted sesame seeds

Direction

- Set an outdoor grill to medium heat and start preheating. Glaze the grate lightly with oil.

- Use a brush to glaze 1 tablespoon of oil on both sides of nopales. Sprinkle with salt and pepper to taste. Place on the preheated grill and cook, flipping half way through, for 7 to 9 minutes or until nopales become soft. Remove from grill and allow it to cool until safe to handle. Cut nopales into 1/2 inch strips.

- On a serving plate, place onion, serrano chiles and tomatoes in layers. Place grilled nopales on top of vegetables bed; sprinkle salad with remaining 2 tablespoons oil and lime juice. Add oregano and cilantro on top. Put in cotija cheese.

- Cut each avocado half without removing the skin; gently scoop sliced avocado on top of the salad in a fan shape using a spoon. Add sesame seeds and additional salt and pepper on top.

Nutrition Information

Calories: 335 calories;

Total Carbohydrate: 17.4

Cholesterol: 7

Protein: 5.5

Total Fat: 29.5

Sodium: 844

Escarole Siciliano

Serving: 3

Ingredients

3 tablespoons olive oil

2 medium heads escarole - rinsed, dried and chopped

1/2 cup lemon juice

2 tablespoons capers

1 pinch salt

10 kalamata olives

ground black pepper to taste

Direction

In a wok, heat oil over high heat. Put in escarole; cook and stir until greens turn wilted. Add lemon juice, stir well. Add olives, salt and carpers; cook and stir well for another 15 seconds. Add salt and black pepper to season. Serve immediately.

Nutrition Information

Calories: 224 calories;

Cholesterol: 0

Protein: 4.8

Total Fat: 17.5

Sodium: 450

Total Carbohydrate: 16.4

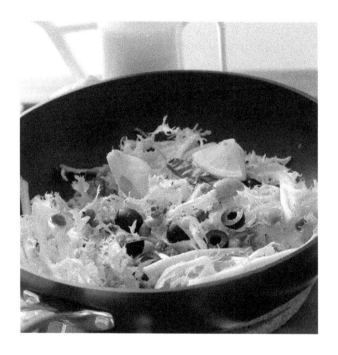

Fall Salad With Quinoa, Brussels Sprouts, And Pomegranate

Serving: 4

Ingredients

- 1 tablespoon butter

- 1 1/2 cups quinoa, rinsed and drained

- 1 1/2 cups vegetable broth

- 3 cups roughly chopped Brussels sprouts

- 6 tablespoons olive oil, divided

- salt and ground black pepper to taste

- 1/3 cup white wine vinegar

- 1/4 cup honey

- 2 tablespoons Dijon mustard

- 1 clove garlic, minced

- 1 pinch herbes de Provence, or to taste

- 4 cups arugula

- 1 1/4 cups pomegranate seeds

- 1/3 cup roasted and salted shelled pistachios

- 1/2 cup crumbled goat cheese

- 4 slices multigrain bread, toasted

Direction

Let butter melt over medium-high heat in a small pot. Toss in quinoa and sauté for 1-3 minutes, until quinoa starts to pop and brown. Pour in broth. Put lid on. Lower the heat to low. Let it simmer for 25-minutes, until all the water is gone.

Set the oven to preheat at 400F (200C). Prepare a baking sheet with parchment paper.

Meanwhile, arrange the Brussel sprouts on the baking sheet. Drizzle 2 tablespoons of olive oil on. Sprinkle on salt and pepper. Toss to coat well.

Roast the Brussel sprouts for 15-20 minutes in the oven, until brown and cooked through but still firm.

Combine remaining olive oil, honey, vinegar, mustard, salt, pepper, garlic, and herbes de Provence in a bowl.

Mix the roasted Brussel sprouts, cooked quinoa, pistachios, and dressing in a bowl. Toss in 2/3 of the pomegranate seeds, 2/3 of goat cheese, and arugula. Mix gently.

Divide into 4 portions. Top with the rest of the goat cheese and pomegranate seeds. Pair each serving with a slice of toasted bread.

Nutrition Information

Calories: 764 calories;

Total Carbohydrate: 91.4

Cholesterol: 24

Total Fat: 38.3

Protein: 20.8

Sodium: 702

Fennel And Orange Salad

Serving: 4

Ingredients

1 bulb fennel, trimmed and sliced

2 large oranges, sliced into rounds

1 tablespoon olive oil

1 tablespoon red wine vinegar

1 teaspoon poppy seeds

salt to taste

2 bunches arugula - rinsed, dried and chopped

Direction

- In a large bowl, place in fennel and orange. Add in vinegar and olive oil; drizzle salt and poppyseeds.

- Allow to chill, put mixture over a bed of arugula and serve

Nutrition Information

Calories: 128 calories;

Total Fat: 4.7

Sodium: 65

Total Carbohydrate: 20.2

Cholesterol: 0

Protein: 4.9

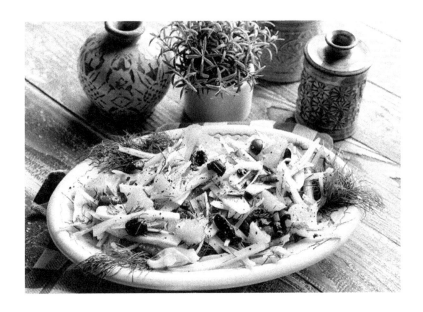

Fennel And Watercress Salad

Serving: 20

Ingredients

1/2 cup chopped dried cranberries

1/4 cup red wine vinegar

1/4 cup balsamic vinegar

1 tablespoon minced garlic

1 1/4 teaspoons salt

1 cup extra virgin olive oil

6 bunches watercress - rinsed, dried and trimmed

3 bulbs fennel - trimmed, cored and thinly sliced

3 small heads radicchio, cored and chopped

1 cup pecan halves, toasted

Direction

- Combine salt, garlic, balsamic vinegar, red wine vinegar and cranberries in a bowl. Add olive oil, whisk well.

- Combine pecans, radicchio, fennel and watercress in a large salad bowl. Mix well the vinaigrette and pour on top of salad. Toss until well coated and serve at once.

Nutrition Information

- Calories: 178 calories;

- Total Fat: 15.4

- Sodium: 202

- Total Carbohydrate: 8.9

- Cholesterol: 0

- Protein: 3.1

French Lentil Salad With Goat Cheese

Serving: 4

Ingredients

3 tablespoons sherry vinegar

3 tablespoons olive oil

1/2 teaspoon minced garlic

1 tablespoon olive oil

1 cup French green lentils

1 (14.5 ounce) can chicken broth

1 cup water

1/3 cup chopped fresh chives

1/4 cup chopped fresh cilantro

1/2 cup crumbled chevre (goat cheese)

1/2 cup quartered grape tomatoes (optional)

Direction

- In a jar that comes with a lid, combine minced garlic, 3 tablespoons olive oil and sherry vinegar in the jar, cover and shake until ingredients are well blended. Set aside.

- In a saucepan, place 1 tablespoon of olive oil, water, chicken broth and lentils, bring mixture to a boil. Cover saucepan with lid, lower the heat to low and simmer for about 20 minutes or until lentils are soft to the bite. Remember not to overcook. Remove from the heat, drain off water and allow it to cool for a minimum of 30 minutes. Move cooled lentils to a mixing bowl.

- Add cilantro, chives and the dressing, stir until well mixed. If the salad needs to be served right away, put in tomatoes and goat cheese. If not, keep salad in the refrigerator and put in tomatoes and goat cheese right before serving.

Nutrition Information

- Calories: 329 calories;

- Protein: 14.7

- Total Fat: 19.5

- Sodium: 533

- Total Carbohydrate: 24.9

- Cholesterol: 16

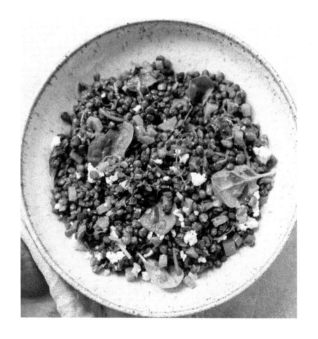

Fresh Avocado Burrata Salad

Serving: 4

Ingredients

- 1 (5 ounce) package baby arugula

- 4 ounces prosciutto, torn into small pieces

- 1/4 cup olive oil

- 1 tablespoon balsamic vinegar

- 1 (4 ounce) ball burrata cheese

- 1 large avocado - peeled, pitted, and sliced

- 1 small Roma tomato, diced

- salt and ground black pepper to taste

Direction

In a bowl, toss together balsamic vinegar, olive oil, prosciutto and baby arugula. Use tongs to move mixture to a large serving plate. Put a ball of burrata cheese in the center. Lay out avocado slices around the plate and place tomato on top. Drizzle with salt and ground black pepper.

Quarter burrata cheese and distribute salad into 4 plates to serve.

Nutrition Information

Calories: 431 calories;

Total Carbohydrate: 8.4

Cholesterol: 45

Protein: 11.9

Total Fat: 39.2

Sodium: 674

Coffee Crusted Hanger Steak With Apple, Fennel, And Herb Salad

Serving: 4

Ingredients

- Coffee Chile Spice Rub:

- 1 tablespoon fennel seeds

- 1 tablespoon cumin seeds

- 1 tablespoon coriander seeds

- 1/4 cup finely ground dark roast coffee beans

- 1/4 cup ground ancho chile pepper

- 1/4 cup brown sugar

- 2 1/2 tablespoons kosher salt

- 2 tablespoons hot smoked paprika

- 2 teaspoons ground black pepper

- 2 teaspoons red pepper flakes
- Steak:
- 1 pound hanger steak
- salt to taste
- 1 teaspoon olive oil
- 4 shallots, halved
- 3 cloves garlic, smashed
- 3 sprigs fresh thyme
- 1 tablespoon butter, cut in small pieces
- Salad Dressing:
- 1 lemon, zested and juiced
- 1 tablespoon olive oil
- 2 teaspoons honey
- salt and ground black pepper to taste
- Salad:
- 1 bulb fennel, halved
- 1/2 lemon, juiced

- 1/2 apple, cut into matchstick-size pieces

- 1 tablespoon fresh mint leaves, or to taste

- 1 tablespoon fresh parsley leaves, or to taste

- 1 tablespoon fresh cilantro leaves, or to taste

- 1/4 cup pomegranate seeds

- 2 tablespoons chopped hazelnuts

Direction

- In a skillet over medium-high heat, put in coriander seeds, cumin seeds and fennel seeds, cook and stir for 1 to 2 minutes until toasted and scented. Move to a food processor or spice grinder; add in red pepper flakes, black pepper, paprika, kosher salt, brown sugar, ancho chile pepper and coffee. Grind until spice rub mixture achieves a medium-coarse texture.

- Cut steak into 4-ounce pieces. Use a knife to lightly score steak into 1/2 inch-1/2 inch. Add salt to season. Use spice rub to rub the steak. Set to medium-high and start heating a cast iron skillet. Make sure the spice rub is packed onto all sides of the steak, place the steak in the hot cast iron skillet; pour about 1 teaspoon of olive oil over steak.

- Cook steak for about 4 minutes until well browned in the cast iron skillet. Turn the steak over and scatter butter, thyme, smashed garlic and shallots in the skillet around steak. Cook for 4 to 5 minutes more until steak reaches the doneness you want. Use an instant-read thermometer to measure the temperature of steak, it should be inserted in the middle and read at least 140°F (60°C). Allow steak to rest for 5 minutes then cut it into thin slices.

- In a small bowl, whisk together salt, pepper, honey, olive oil, lemon zest and juice of 1 lemon until mixed evenly.

- In a bowl, add in thinly shave fennel and juice of 1/2 lemon, toss well to preserve color. Add cilantro, parsley, mint and apple. Pour dressing over salad, mixed gently until well coated; add salt and pepper to season. Place steak slices on

top of salad and scatter hazelnuts,
pomegranate seeds and roasted shallots on top.

Nutrition Information

- Calories: 413 calories;

- Sodium: 3782

- Total Carbohydrate: 53.9

- Cholesterol: 33

- Protein: 20.7

- Total Fat: 17.1

Mango Papaya Salad

Serving: 6

Ingredients

1 large mango - peeled, seeded and halved

1 medium papaya - peeled, seeded and halved

1 avocado - peeled, pitted and diced

3 tablespoons balsamic vinegar

1 tablespoon butter

1/4 cup blanched slivered almonds

1 teaspoon brown sugar

1 head romaine lettuce, torn into bite-size pieces

salt to taste

Direction

- Put half of the papaya and half of the mango into the container of a blender or food processor together with balsamic vinegar. Blend until it turns smooth, and reserve.

- Put butter in a small skillet to melt on medium heat. Put in almonds and cook stirring continuously until lightly browned. Mix in brown sugar and stir to coat. Separate from heat, and place candied almonds onto a piece of waxed paper, getting rid of any clumps. Reserve to cool.

- Just prior to serving, put romaine lettuce in a large serving bowl. Then cube leftover papaya halves and mango, and gently toss with lettuce and avocado. Drizzle on the pureed fruit over the salad and lightly salt. Sprinkle with candied almonds, and serve right away.

Nutrition Information

- Calories: 148 calories;

- Total Carbohydrate: 16

- Cholesterol: 5

- Protein: 2.7

- Total Fat: 9.4

- Sodium: 25

Mandarin Orange Salad

Serving: 6

Ingredients

- Dressing
- 1 onion, minced
- 2/3 cup white sugar
- 1 tablespoon dry mustard
- 1 teaspoon celery seed
- 1 teaspoon black pepper
- 1/2 cup distilled white vinegar
- 1/2 cup olive oil
- Salad
- 1 head romaine lettuce, chopped
- 1 (10 ounce) can mandarin oranges, drained
- 5 ounces fresh mushrooms, sliced

- 3 tablespoons slivered almonds

- 3 tablespoons crumbled cooked bacon

Direction

- In a small bowl, place black pepper, celery seed, mustard, sugar and onion. Stir in vinegar to dissolve the sugar. Add olive oil and whisk till the dressing is thickened. Cover and store for at least 3 hours in the fridge.

- For the salad, in a large bowl, toss bacon, almonds, mushrooms, oranges and lettuce together. Drizzle dressing over and toss again till coated.

Nutrition Information

- Calories: 332 calories;

- Sodium: 120

- Total Carbohydrate: 34.1

- Cholesterol: 2

- Protein: 4.6

- Total Fat: 21.2

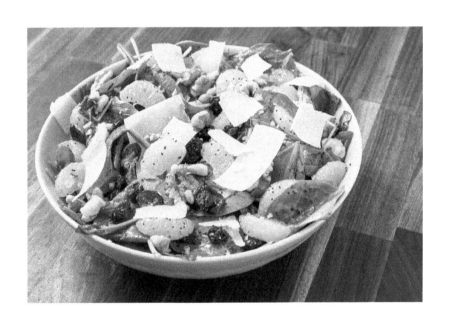

Gourmet Tuna Salad

Serving: 4

Ingredients

- 1 (12 ounce) can albacore tuna in water, drained and flaked

- 2 green onions, chopped

- 1 stalk celery, diced

- 1/4 cup pimento-stuffed green olives, chopped

- 2 tablespoons capers, chopped

- 1/4 cup blanched slivered almonds

- 1 dash Worcestershire sauce

- 1/2 cup mayonnaise

- 1/4 cup sour cream

Direction

- Combine almonds, capers, green olives, celery, green onions and tuna in a mixing bowl

- Whisk together Worcestershire sauce, sour cream and mayonnaise in a small bowl

- Mix together tuna mixture and dressing. Place mixture over bed of lettuce or with croissant as a tuna salad sandwich, and serve

Nutrition Information

- Calories: 396 calories;

- Total Fat: 32.4

- Sodium: 908

- Total Carbohydrate: 4.1

- Cholesterol: 52

- Protein: 22.5

Calamari Salad

Serving: 12

Ingredients

2 lemons, juiced

6 cloves garlic, peeled and minced

1 sprig fresh parsley, chopped

salt and pepper to taste

3 pounds squid, cleaned and sliced into rounds

1 (2.25 ounce) can pitted black olives

4 stalks celery, chopped

Direction

- Mix parsley, garlic, and lemon juice in a medium bowl. Season with pepper and salt.

- Boil a medium pot of water. Mix in squid. Cook until tender for about 3 minutes. Drain.

- Toss lemon juice mixture, celery, olives, and squid. Cover and keep in fridge to chill. Serve.

Nutrition Information

Calories: 119 calories;

Cholesterol: 264

Protein: 18.2

Total Fat: 2.2

Sodium: 108

Total Carbohydrate: 6.8

Greek Pasta Salad With Roasted Vegetables And Feta

Serving: 6

Ingredients

1 red bell pepper, cut into 1/2 inch pieces

1 yellow bell pepper, chopped

1 medium eggplant, cubed

3 small yellow squash, cut in 1/4 inch slices

6 tablespoons extra virgin olive oil

1/4 teaspoon salt

1/4 teaspoon ground black pepper

1 1/2 ounces sun-dried tomatoes, soaked in 1/2 cup boiling water

1/2 cup torn arugula leaves

1/2 cup chopped fresh basil

2 tablespoons balsamic vinegar

2 tablespoons minced garlic

4 ounces crumbled feta cheese

1 (12 ounce) package farfalle pasta

Direction

- Preheat oven to 230°C/450°F. Line foil on cookie sheet; spray using nonstick cooking spray.

- Toss 2 tbsp. olive oil, pepper, salt, squash, eggplant, and yellow and red bell pepper in medium bowl. Put on prepped cookie sheet.

- In preheated oven, bake veggies for 25 minutes till lightly browned, occasionally tossing.

- Cook pasta in big pot with salted boiling water till al dente for 10-12 minutes; drain.

- Drain softened sun-dried tomatoes; keep water. Toss basil, arugula, sun-drained tomatoes, cooked pasta and roasted veggies in big bowl. Mix feta cheese, garlic, balsamic vinegar, reserved water from tomatoes and leftover olive oil in. Toss till coated. Season to taste with pepper and salt; immediately serve or refrigerate till chilled.

Nutrition Information

- Calories: 446 calories;

- Protein: 13.8

- Total Fat: 19.5

- Sodium: 324

- Total Carbohydrate: 56.9

- Cholesterol: 17

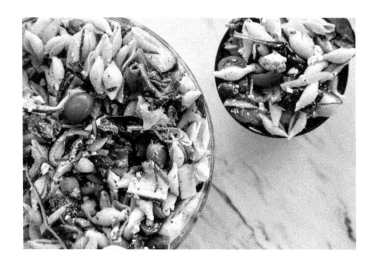

Green Apple Salad With Blueberries, Feta, And Walnuts

Serving: 4

Ingredients

- 4 cups mixed salad greens such as leaf lettuce, endive, and radicchio

- 1 large Granny Smith, cut into small cubes

- 1/2 cup chopped walnuts

- 1/2 cup crumbled feta cheese

- 1/2 cup dried cranberries

- 2 tablespoons finely chopped green onions (optional)

- Dressing:

- 1/4 cup vegetable oil

- 1/4 cup blueberries

- 2 tablespoons extra-virgin olive oil

- 2 tablespoons balsamic vinegar

- 1/4 teaspoon salt

Direction

- In a big bowl, put a layer of green onions, cranberries, feta cheese, walnuts, Granny smith apple, and salad greens.

- In a blender or a food processor, mix salt, balsamic vinegar, extra-virgin olive oil, blueberries, and vegetable oil together, pulse into a creamy dressing.

- Put the dressing on the salad, mix to coat. Refrigerate until ready to serve.

Nutrition Information

- Calories: 417 calories;

- Total Fat: 34.3

- Sodium: 372

- Total Carbohydrate: 26.1

Green Mango Salad

Serving: 4

Ingredients

1 pound green mangoes - peeled, pitted, and cut into matchsticks

1/2 large red onion, thinly sliced

1 large ripe avocado, peeled and cut into wedges

2 tablespoons chopped dry-roasted peanuts

1 tablespoon soy sauce

1 tablespoon white sugar

1 tablespoon lime juice

1 teaspoon Thai pepper sauce

1 clove garlic

Direction

- In a large bowl, mix together peanuts, avocado, onion and mangoes

- In a small bowl, combine garlic, Thai pepper sauce, lime juice, sugar and soy sauce. Pour dressing over mango mixture. Stir properly until well coated

- Allow to sit at room temperature for 10 minutes in order that the flavors combined well then serve

Nutrition Information

- Calories: 236 calories;

- Sodium: 324

- Total Carbohydrate: 32.1

- Cholesterol: 0

- Protein: 3.5

- Total Fat: 12.8

Green Salad With Cranberry Vinaigrette

Serving: 8

Ingredients

1 cup sliced almonds

3 tablespoons red wine vinegar

1/3 cup olive oil

1/4 cup fresh cranberries

1 tablespoon Dijon mustard

1/2 teaspoon minced garlic

1/2 teaspoon salt

1/2 teaspoon ground black pepper

2 tablespoons water

1/2 red onion, thinly sliced

4 ounces crumbled blue cheese

1 pound mixed salad greens

Direction

- Preheat the oven to 190°C or 375°Fahrenheit. In a single layer, place almonds on a baking sheet. Toast almonds in the oven for five minutes until it starts to brown.

- Process water, vinegar, pepper, oil, salt, cranberries, garlic, and mustard in a food processor or blender until smooth.

- Mix greens, almonds, blue cheese, onion, and the vinegar mixture together in a large bowl until well coated.

Nutrition Information

- Calories: 218 calories;

- Total Carbohydrate: 6.2

- Cholesterol: 11

- Protein: 6.5

- Total Fat: 19.2

- Sodium: 405

Grilled Panzanella Salad With Peaches And Fennel

Serving: 4

Ingredients

- 1 large shallot, sliced thin

- 2 tablespoons white wine vinegar

- 1 teaspoon maple syrup (or sweetener of choice)

- 1/2 teaspoon fine sea salt and fresh pepper

- 6 tablespoons extra-virgin olive oil, divided

- 1 clove garlic

- 4 slices hearty bread

- 2 peaches, sliced into wedges

- 2 cups baby arugula

- 1 cup torn basil leaves

- 1 large fennel bulb, halved, cored and thinly shaved on a mandoline

- Reynolds Wrap® Non Stick Aluminum Foil

Direction

- Prepare Reynolds Wrap(R) Non Stick Aluminum Foil, cut a large piece and fit it firmly to the grill grate. Set the grill to medium heat

- While waiting the grill to heat, make the dressing. In a shallow bowl, add maple syrup, vinegar and shallot, season with a couple pinches of salt and pepper. Allow to sit for about 10 minutes until shallots become soft. Add in 4 tablespoon of the oil, whisk properly until dressing is blended and mixed. Set aside.

- Use a knife to cut garlic clove in half. Gently rub the cut side of the garlic to both sides of each slice of bread. Lightly glaze each side of the bread with 1 tablespoon of oil.

- Place bread on the heated grill and cook for about 7 to 10 minutes until bread becomes firm and toasted. Remove from the grill and allow to cool.

- Use the brush to glaze peaches with the remaining tablespoon of oil, season with a couple pinches of salt. On the foil-covered grill, place the peaches and cook for about 4 to 5 minutes until it turns light brown and firm. Remove from the heat and set aside.

- Mix together basil and arugula in a large serving bowl. Rip the bread in to large chunks, add into the bowl. Add in fennel and peaches. Add in the dressing, mix well then toss thoroughly

Nutrition Information

Calories: 289 calories;

Total Fat: 21.3

Sodium: 410

Total Carbohydrate: 21.7

Cholesterol: 0

Protein: 3.2

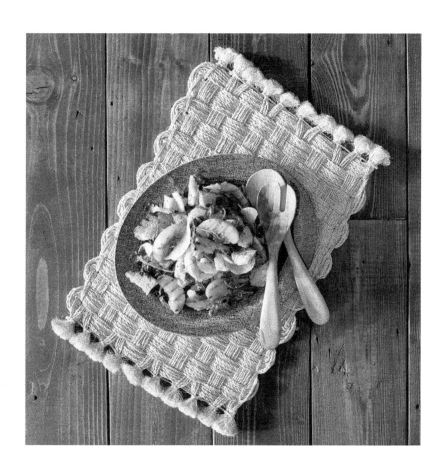

Grilled Romaine Salad

Serving: 8

Ingredients

1/2 cup olive oil

3 tablespoons white sugar

1 teaspoon dried rosemary

1 teaspoon dried thyme

1/4 teaspoon salt

1/4 teaspoon ground black pepper

8 Roma (plum) tomatoes, halved lengthwise

2 shallots, halved lengthwise and peeled

1/2 cup balsamic vinegar

2 tablespoons brown sugar

1 3/4 cups olive oil

4 romaine hearts

1 tablespoon olive oil

salt and pepper to taste

Direction

- Preheat the oven to 225°F (110°C). In a big Ziplock plastic bag, combine the thyme, olive oil, pepper, salt, rosemary and white sugar together. Put in the tomatoes then seal the Ziplock bag and shake well until fully coated. Place the coated halved tomatoes on a baking sheet, cut-side up. Put in the preheated oven and let it bake for 2 1/2 hours. Remove the tomatoes from the oven and allow it to cool down.

- Chop the shallots finely using a food processor or a blender. Put in the brown sugar and vinegar and blend until the consistency is smooth. While frequently blending, put in 1 3/4 cups of oil gradually until the mixture has thickened.

- Preheat the grill to high heat. Use a brush to coat the romaine hearts with 1 tablespoon of olive oil then sprinkle it with pepper and salt to taste.

- Put the seasoned romaine hearts onto the preheated grill. Let it cook on the grill for 5-10 minutes while turning it from time to time until the romaine hearts are burnt a little bit but not completely heated through. Serve it on salad plates while warm with the tomato pieces arranged around the salad; pour the shallot dressing on top.

Nutrition Information

Calories: 622 calories;

Total Fat: 62.8

Sodium: 87

Total Carbohydrate: 16.6

Cholesterol: 0

Protein: 1.5

Ham And Swiss Salad With Red Currants

Serving: 6

Ingredients

1 head romaine lettuce, rinsed, patted dry and chopped

4 ounces arugula, washed and dried

4 ounces sliced mushrooms

1 cup grape tomatoes, halved

1 shallot, thinly sliced

1 cup fresh red currants

1/2 cup shredded Swiss cheese

4 ounces honey ham, chopped

1/4 cup balsamic vinegar

1/4 cup extra virgin olive oil

salt and pepper to taste

Direction

- In a large salad bowl, mix together ham, Swiss cheese, currants, shallot, tomatoes, mushrooms, arugula and romaine. In a small bowl, put in salt and pepper, olive oil and balsamic vinegar, whisk until mixed well. Pour the dressing over the salad and toss until well coated.

Nutrition Information

- Calories: 187 calories;

- Total Fat: 12.8

- Sodium: 188

- Total Carbohydrate: 11.3

- Cholesterol: 18

- Protein: 8.1

Hot Chicken Liver And Fennel Salad

Serving: 4

Ingredients

- 4 cups spinach, rinsed and chopped

- 1 bulb fennel - trimmed, quartered and sliced

- 2 tablespoons butter

- 1/4 cup olive oil

- 2 cloves garlic, minced

- 1 pound chicken livers, trimmed and sliced

- 1/2 cup chicken broth

- 1 teaspoon capers, chopped

- 4 anchovy filets, rinsed and chopped

- 1 teaspoon dried sage

- 1/2 teaspoon salt

- 1/4 teaspoon ground black pepper

Direction

- Separate spinach into 4 salad plates

- Melt 1 tablespoon butter in a large deep skillet over medium heat; add in fennel, cook for about 3 minutes or until it becomes soft. Remove fennel from skillet, set aside

- Heat olive oil with remaining butter in the same skillet; add in garlic, cook for 1 minute. Add in chicken livers; cook for 3 to 4 minutes or until the liver is no longer pink in the center.

- Return cooked fennel to skillet. Add in salt and pepper, sage, carpers, anchovies and stock; cook the mixture over high heat for 2 to 3 minutes or until the amount of sauce is slightly decreased

- Add a spoon of mixture over each salad dish and decorate with fennel leaves. Serve immediately

Nutrition Information

- Calories: 348 calories;

- Cholesterol: 411

- Protein: 23.5

- Total Fat: 25.7

- Sodium: 831

- Total Carbohydrate: 6.3

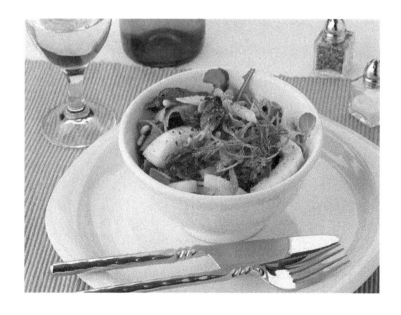

Jarjeer (Arugula) Salad

Serving: 4

Ingredients

- 1 bunch arugula

- 2 onions, thinly sliced

- 1 cup chopped mushrooms

- 1 tomato, diced (optional)

- 1 teaspoon extra virgin olive oil

- 1/2 lemon, juiced

- 2 teaspoons sumac (see Note)

- Salt to taste

Direction

- Wash arugula leaves and then dry.

- Spread the leaves onto a large plate and then spread a layer of tomato, onions, and mushrooms.

- Whisk sumac, olive oil, and lemon juice together.

- Add salt to taste and spread atop the salad.

Nutrition Information

- Calories: 62 calories;

- Protein: 3.2

- Total Fat: 1.8

- Sodium: 22

- Total Carbohydrate: 10.4

- Cholesterol: 0

GOURMET
RECIPES
FOR
BEGINNERS

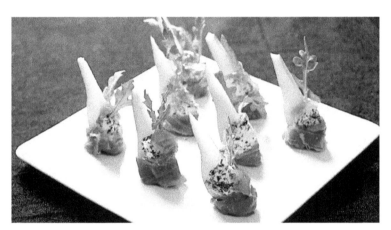

APPETIZERS

IMPROVISE YOURSELF AS A STARRED CHEF

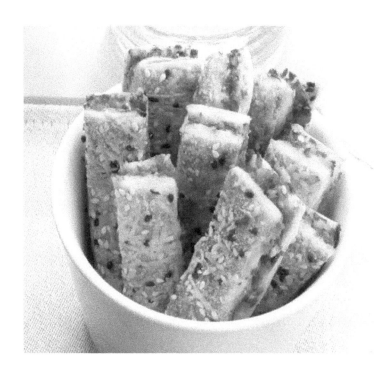

Mussels Vinaigrette

Serving: 6

Ingredients

- 1/4 cup red wine vinegar

- 2 tablespoons chopped fresh parsley

- 1 hard-cooked egg, chopped

- 24 fresh mussels, scrubbed and debearded

- 1 small green bell pepper, seeded and diced

- 1 small red bell pepper, seeded and diced

- 1 small yellow bell peppers, seeded and diced

- 1/2 cup olive oil

- 1/2 teaspoon salt

- 1 pinch ground black pepper

Direction

- In a big pot, boil an-inch of water. Put the mussels, place cover, and allow to steam for 3 to 5 minutes, till all are open. Let drain. Take off one side of every shell, and on a serving platter, set mussels with open shell. Throw any mussels that remain closed.

- Combine together the pepper, salt, egg, parsley, wine vinegar, olive oil, and red, yellow and green bell peppers in a medium bowl. Scoop on top of mussels on shells. Chill till serving.

Nutrition Information

- Calories: 240 calories;
- Total Fat: 20.4
- Sodium: 389
- Total Carbohydrate: 5.5
- Cholesterol: 53
- Protein: 9.1

Olive Bread Crostini With Red Pepper Spread

Serving: 12

Ingredients

- 1 small garlic, minced

- 1/2 teaspoon salt

- 1 (12 ounce) jar roasted red peppers, drained and dried with a paper towel

- 3 tablespoons olive oil, divided

- 2 tablespoons chopped fresh basil

- 1 1/2 teaspoons balsamic vinegar

- 1/2 teaspoon packed brown sugar

- 1/4 teaspoon ground black pepper

- 12 (1/4 inch thick) slices olive bread, halved diagonally

Direction

- Mash salt and garlic together into a paste using a pestle and mortar; move to a food processor. Add 1 tablespoon oil and roasted red peppers; pulse until the mixture turn to a coarse puree. Pour red pepper spread in a bowl and stir in pepper, sugar, vinegar and basil.

- Set the oven to 350°F (175°C) and start preheating.

- Brush remaining 2 tablespoons oil on both sides of bread slices. Place bread in a single layer on a baking sheet.

- Place bread slices in the preheated oven and bake for about 25 minutes or until golden, remember to flip one time while baking. Place crostini on a rack to cool.

- Place 3/4 tablespoon red pepper spread on top of each crostini right before serving.

Nutrition Information

- Calories: 56 calories;

- Cholesterol: 0

- Protein: 0.9

- Total Fat: 3.7

- Sodium: 521

- Total Carbohydrate: 5

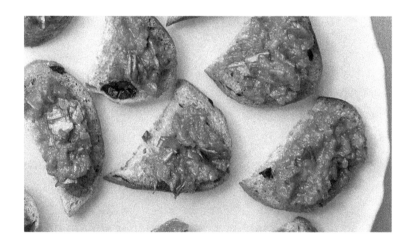

Olive Puffs

Serving: 12

Ingredients

- 24 pimento-stuffed green olives

- 1 (17.25 ounce) package frozen puff pastry, thawed

Direction

- Set the oven to 400°F (200°C), and start preheating.

- Slice pastry into strips of about 1/2-inch wide and 6 inches long. Wrap each olive with a belt of pastry. Put on unoiled baking sheet.

- Bake in the oven for 20 minutes, until golden brown.

Nutrition Information

- Calories: 230 calories;

- Total Fat: 16.2

- Sodium: 265

- Total Carbohydrate: 18.3

- Cholesterol: 0

- Protein: 3

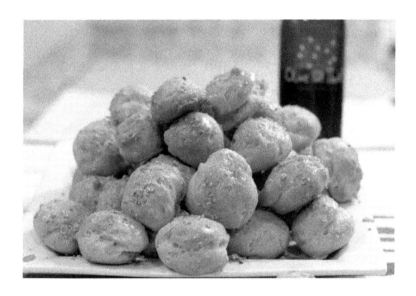

Parmesan Thyme Crisps

Serving: 15

Ingredients

- 8 ounces freshly grated Parmesan cheese
- 4 teaspoons fresh thyme leaves

Direction

- Prepare oven by preheating it to 300° F (150° C). Place parchment paper on 2 baking sheets.

- Mix thyme leaves and Parmesan cheese in a bowl. Drop big teaspoonfuls of the mixture on the lined baking sheets, keeping them 2 inches away from each other. Use your fingers to lightly press and flatten them to create circles that are 2 inches in diameter.

- Place in the preheated and bake for 8-10 minutes until crisp and slightly brown. Slightly cool for 2 minutes on baking sheets. Use a spatula to loosen the edges and lift from the parchment paper. Move to wire racks and completely cool for 10 minutes until firm.

Nutrition Information

- Calories: 65 calories;

- Total Fat: 4.3

- Sodium: 231

- Total Carbohydrate: 0.7

- Cholesterol: 13

- Protein: 5.8

Pate Recipe

Serving: 24

Ingredients

- 1 pound bacon strips, diced

- 3 medium onions, chopped

- 3 cloves garlic

- 1 pound chicken livers, trimmed and chopped

- 1 pound veal, trimmed and cubed

- 1 cup heavy cream

- 1/2 cup milk

- 3/4 cup butter

- 1 pinch salt and pepper to taste

Direction

- Place a large skillet pan on the stove and turn on to medium-high heat then put the bacon in. Let it cook until dried up, then stir in the whole garlic cloves and onion. Continue to stir and cook until onion become soft. Put in the veal cubes and chicken livers to the skillet, let it cook until the pink color faded. Let it cool aside.

- Get a 9x5 inch loaf pan or mold and use a waxed paper to line it, or use a cooking spray then put aside. Prepare a food processor and place in the container the meat mixture, then blend until chopped into small pieces. Do not turn it into a liquid. Then place a large skillet on the stove and turn on to medium heat and put the butter in to melt. Stir in the meat mixture, and add in the milk and heavy cream. Let it cook until warmed enough. Put pepper and salt to taste, then transfer into the mold or loaf pan. Let it chill in the refrigerator for 4 hours until serving time.

Nutrition Information

- Calories: 178 calories;

- Total Fat: 14.2

- Sodium: 214

- Total Carbohydrate: 2.2

- Cholesterol: 155

- Protein: 10.1

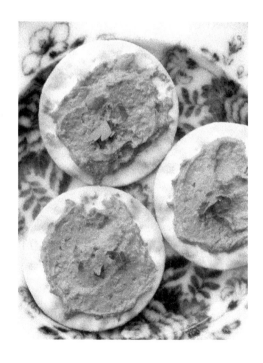

Peaches With Burrata, Basil, And Raspberry Balsamic Syrup

Serving: 4

Ingredients

- 1 (4 ounce) ball Burrata cheese, at room temperature

- 1 peach, sliced

- 1 tablespoon thinly sliced fresh basil leaves

- 2 tablespoons extra-virgin olive oil

- 3 tablespoons raspberry balsamic vinegar

- flaked sea salt

- freshly ground black pepper (optional)

Direction

Expose the soft and creamy core of the Burrata cheese by carefully tearing it open then place it in the center of a plate. Set the slices of peach around and all over the cheese then drizzle it with basil leaves, topping it off with olive oil.

Put the raspberry balsamic vinegar in a small saucepan and wait for it to boil then lower down the heat to medium-low and let it simmer for 5 minutes or until the vinegar has turned into a thick syrup. Using a spoon, take some of the balsamic syrup and dribble it over the peaches and cheese then add flavor by seasoning it with black pepper and sea salt.

Nutrition Information

- Calories: 159 calories;
- Protein: 4.1
- Total Fat: 12.8
- Sodium: 176
- Total Carbohydrate: 3.9
- Cholesterol: 20

Perfect Pot Stickers

Serving: 6

Ingredients

- Filling:

- 1 pound ground pork

- 4 cloves minced garlic

- 1/2 cup finely chopped green onions

- 3 tablespoons very finely minced fresh ginger

- 2 tablespoons soy sauce

- 1 teaspoon soy sauce

- 1 teaspoon sesame oil

- 1 pinch cayenne pepper

- 1 1/2 cups finely chopped green cabbage

- Dough:

- 2 1/2 cups all-purpose flour

- 3/4 teaspoon kosher salt

- 1 cup hot water, about 130 -150 F (55-65 C)

- Dipping Sauce:

- 1/4 cup seasoned rice vinegar

- 1/4 cup soy sauce

- For Frying:

- 6 tablespoons vegetable oil for frying, or as needed - divided

- 8 tablespoons water for steaming, divided

Direction

In a mixing bowl, combine the ground pork, ginger, garlic, green onions, sesame oil, 2 tablespoons + 1 teaspoon soy sauce, and cayenne then top this with chopped green cabbage. Using a fork, mix all of them together until well blended. Lightly press together then cover it with plastic. Keep it refrigerated for about 1 hour until it has chilled.

In a mixing bowl, combine the kosher salt and flour then gradually add hot water. Using a wooden spoon, stir together until the mixture has formed a rough dough. Cover your hands with flour and then move the dough to a work surface. Knead the dough for about 3-5 minutes until it's become smooth and pliable. Just drizzle with a little flour if the dough gets a bit sticky. Using a plastic wrap, wrap the dough and leave it for 30 minutes to rest.

Divide the dough into 4 equal parts when it has rested. Use a dishcloth to cover the 3 parts while you are working on the first part of dough. Roll each dough into a small log about 3/4 inch, around the thickness of a thumb. Each log should be divided into 6 equal parts then each part should be formed into pot sticker wrappers by rolling each into about 3 1/2-inch thin circle on a surface that's been lightly floured. Do this to all the remaining dough pieces.

Wet your finger to lightly moisten a wrapper's edges. Scoop a small part of the ground pork mixture and place it onto a wrapper's center. Fold the 2 sides of the wrapper up and pinch it together in the center. Create pleats along one side of the wrapper by pinching together the remaining edges. Flatten the bottom of the pot sticker by lightly tapping it on the work surface and make a slight curve in the sticker to make sure it stands upright in the pan. Move the pot sticker to a plate that's been well-floured and repeat the process with the rest of the dough and filling.

Combine the soy sauce and seasoned rice vinegar in a small mixing bowl. This will be the dipping sauce for the dumplings.

Place a cooking pan over medium-high heat and heat the oil in the pan. Put around 6-7 potstickers in the oil with its flat side down. Cook the potstickers for about 2 minutes, until the bottoms are golden brown. Sprinkle with some water and cover the pan immediately then leave it to steam for 3 minutes. Uncover the pan and lower the heat to medium. Cook for 1-2 minutes more, until the bottoms of the stickers are already brown and crunchy and the water has evaporated. Move the pot stickers to a warm serving bowl or plate. Do the same with the remaining dumplings then serve together with the sauce for dipping.

Petit Toasts With Brie, Fig, And Thyme

Serving: 10

Ingredients

- 1 (2.8 ounce) package toasted baguette slices (such as Trois Petits Cochons® Petits Toasts)

- 1/2 pound Brie cheese, cut into 1-inch squares

- 1 cup fig preserves

- 1/2 cup toasted slivered almonds

- 1 teaspoon balsamic glaze (reduced balsamic vinegar), or more to taste

- 1 pinch fresh thyme, or more to taste

Direction

- On a serving dish, put toasts and put a Brie cheese square on each top. Put fig preserves on the Brie cheese then top with almonds.

Sprinkle over each toast a fine line of balsamic glaze and put thyme on top.

Nutrition Information

- Calories: 132 calories;

- Total Fat: 9.2

- Sodium: 194

- Total Carbohydrate: 5.8

- Cholesterol: 23

- Protein: 6.8

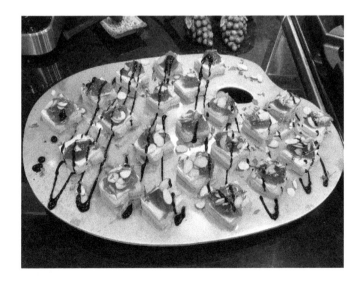

Pita Chips

Serving: 24

Ingredients

- 12 pita bread pockets

- 1/2 cup olive oil

- 1/2 teaspoon ground black pepper

- 1 teaspoon garlic salt

- 1/2 teaspoon dried basil

- 1 teaspoon dried chervil

Direction

- Heat oven to 200 degrees Celsius or 400 degrees Fahrenheit.

- Slice every pita bread to 8 triangles. Put triangles on a lined cookie sheet.

- Mix chervil, basil, salt, pepper, and oil in a small boil. Brush oil mixture on every triangle.

- Bake in oven for 7 minutes until crispy and lightly browned. Watch to avoid burning.

Nutrition Information

- Calories: 125 calories;

- Cholesterol: 0

- Protein: 3.2

- Total Fat: 5.3

- Sodium: 246

- Total Carbohydrate: 17.7

Pork Dumplings

Serving: 6

Ingredients

- 100 (3.5 inch square) wonton wrappers

- 1 3/4 pounds ground pork

- 1 tablespoon minced fresh ginger root

- 4 cloves garlic, minced

- 2 tablespoons thinly sliced green onion

- 4 tablespoons soy sauce

- 3 tablespoons sesame oil

- 1 egg, beaten

- 5 cups finely shredded Chinese cabbage

Direction

- Mix together egg, sesame oil, green onion, ginger, pork, garlic, soy sauce, and cabbage in a large bowl. Stir until well-combined.

- Put a teaspoon-full of pork filling on each wonton skin. Wet the edges with water and seal to form a triangle by folding edges over. Slightly roll the edges to seal in the filling. Leave the dumplings on a lightly-floured surface or container until they are ready to be cooked.

- Cook the dumplings for about 15 to 20 minutes in a covered metal steamer or bamboo steamer. Serve right away.

Nutrition Information

- Calories: 752 calories;

- Total Fat: 28.8

- Sodium: 1449

- Total Carbohydrate: 81.1

- Cholesterol: 129

- Protein: 39.2

Potstickers (Chinese Dumplings)

Serving: 12

Ingredients

- 1 pound raw shrimp, peeled and deveined

- 4 pounds ground beef

- 1 tablespoon minced fresh ginger root

- 1 shallot, minced

- 1 bunch green onions, chopped

- 3 leaves napa cabbage, chopped

- 2 tablespoons soy sauce

- 1 teaspoon Asian (toasted) sesame oil

- salt and white pepper to taste

- 1 pinch white sugar

- 1 (10 ounce) package round gyoza/potsticker wrappers

- vegetable oil

- 1/4 cup water

Direction

- Process the shrimp in the work bowl in a food processor until it's very finely ground. Move it to a large bowl then set it aside. Process the ground beef in the food processor as well until it becomes a fine grind, doing it in batches, then set it aside as well. Mix together the ground beef and shrimp, shallot, ginger, green onions, soy sauce, napa cabbage, sesame oil, white sugar, and salt and pepper until all ingredients are well blended.

- Put a wrapper on a work surface and get a scant teaspoon of the filling then put it in the center of the wrapper to fill the pot stickers. Dip your finger in water to wet it then dampen the wrapper's edges. Enclose the filling by folding the dough into the shape of a half-moon then press and seal the sticker for removing extra air and tightly sealing the edges together. Create a traditional look by folding several small pleats in the wrapper's top half before sealing the filling in. Put the filled wrappers on a baking sheet lined with parchment paper, then refrigerate as you fill and seal the rest of the pot stickers.

- In a big nonstick cooking pan with a lid, heat the oil over medium heat. Fry the pot stickers in the hot oil for 1-2 minutes until the bottoms are golden, the flat sides down and with a few spaces apart so they don't crowd. Turn over the pot stickers then pour water over them. Cover the pan and leave the dumplings to steam for 5-7 minutes until they begin to fry in oil again and the water has nearly evaporated. Uncover the pan and leave the dumplings to cook for another 2-3 minutes, until the wrapper has shrunk tightly onto the filling and all the water has evaporated.

Nutrition Information

- Calories: 411 calories;

- Protein: 34.5

- Total Fat: 22.3

- Sodium: 454

- Total Carbohydrate: 16.1

- Cholesterol: 152

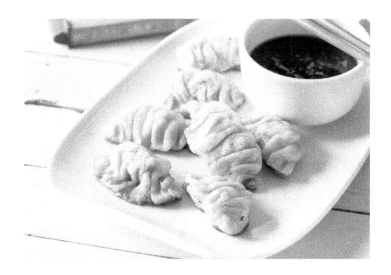

Prosciutto Parmesan And Pine Nut Bruschetta

Serving: 12

Ingredients

- 1 cup butter, softened

- 1 cup diced prosciutto

- 1 cup grated Parmesan cheese

- ground black pepper to taste

- 2 French baguettes, cut into 1/2 inch slices

- 1 cup toasted pine nuts

Direction

- Preheat the oven to 175 °C or 350 °F.

- Cream the butter in a medium bowl. Mix in ground black pepper, Parmesan cheese and prosciutto.

- On a medium baking sheet, put the baguettes. In the preheated oven, heat for 10 minutes till toasted lightly.

- Scatter butter mixture on baguette slices. Set on a big serving plate. Scatter pine nuts over.

Nutrition Information

- Calories: 496 calories;

- Sodium: 949

- Total Carbohydrate: 44.7

- Cholesterol: 58

- Protein: 17.2

- Total Fat: 28.5

Prosciutto And Figs With Goat Cheese

Serving: 8

Ingredients

4 ounces thinly sliced prosciutto

8 dried figs, or as desired

3 ounces goat cheese

Direction

- Warm up oven to 175°C or 350°F.

- On a work surface, lay prosciutto. At the end of each prosciutto slice, place 1 fig. Onto each fig, spread a thin layer of goat cheese. Roll prosciutto around each of the figs and then arrange them on a baking sheet.

- In a preheated oven, bake prosciutto for about 3-4 minutes or until crisp.

Nutrition Information

- Calories: 140 calories;

- Sodium: 331

- Total Carbohydrate: 12.7

- Cholesterol: 21

- Protein: 5.6

- Total Fat: 7.9

Prosciutto And Soppressata Rolls

Serving: 10

Ingredients

- 2 (3 ounce) packages prosciutto

- 1 (.75 ounce) package fresh basil leaves

- 2 (8 ounce) packages fresh mozzarella cheese marinated in olive oil

- toothpicks

- 2 (4 ounce) packages sliced soppressata

Direction

- On a work surface, put a slice of prosciutto, then top it with 1 mozzarella ball and 1 basil leaf.

- Roll the prosciutto around the mozzarella cheese and basil and secure it using a toothpick.

- Redo the process and alternate it with soppressata, until all the ingredients are used up.

- Let it chill in the fridge until ready to serve.

Nutrition Information

- Calories: 281 calories;

- Total Fat: 22

- Sodium: 852

- Total Carbohydrate: 1.9

- Cholesterol: 73

- Protein: 16.8

Quick Fontina Cheese Fondue

Serving: 12

Ingredients

- 1/4 cup butter

- 1/4 cup all-purpose flour

- 1/3 cup dry white wine

- 1/2 teaspoon dry mustard

- 1/4 teaspoon cayenne pepper

- 2 cups heavy whipping cream

- 1/2 cup chicken stock

- 2 cups shredded fontina cheese

Direction

- Place a saucepan on medium heat and melt the butter into it just until a pinch of flour bubbles if you sprinkle it in the oil. Add the flour, whisking it in, until it turns into a thick paste like that of a frosting of a cake. Continue the cooking and the constant whipping for 20 minutes until the flour has goldened and it starts to have the toast-like aroma. Whip in the mustard, wine and the cayenne.

- Add the heavy whipping cream to the flour-butter mixture, whisking it in and continue to cook for 5 minutes, stirring until the sauce has thickened. Toss in the fontina cheese and stir for 1 more minute until the cheese has melted. Pour the sauce into a fondue pot.

Nutrition Information

- Calories: 273 calories;

- Sodium: 259

- Total Carbohydrate: 3.7

- Cholesterol: 90

- Protein: 6.8

- Total Fat: 25.5

Quince Paste

Serving: 32

Ingredients

- 4 1/2 pounds ripe quinces
- 5 1/2 cups white sugar
- water to cover

Direction

Rinse, skin, and remove the core of the quinces; keep the skins and cores. Roughly chop the quinces' flesh and move to a big pan. Use a cheesecloth and kitchen string to wrap the skins and cores; place it in the pan. The pectin in the skin firms up the quince paste.

Pour in just enough water to cover the quinces; boil half-covered for 30-40 minutes until the quinces are very soft. Take out the cheesecloth. Using food mill or sieve, pass the quince flesh through. Avoid using a food processor for it can produce a fine mixture. You should have 2 1/2 lbs of quince pulp.

Move the quince pulp to a pot and add roughly the same amount sugar as the pulp's weight. On low heat, cook and stir until the sugar dissolves. Keep on cooking for 1 1/2 hr until the paste is deep orange and thick; stir regularly using a wooden spoon. Drag the wooden spoon at the base of the pot, the mixture should stick to the wooden spoon and leave a trail.

Line with a greased parchment paper or lightly oil a 9-in x 13-in baking pan. Spread the paste to the baking pan by 1 1/2 -in thick. Smoothen the surface and let it cool.

Let the paste dry in the oven set in the lowest heat not exceeding 52°C or 125°F for 1 1/2 hrs. Cool the paste completely; cut. The traditional European way of drying the paste is by placing it in the cupboard for a week. The leftover juices will evaporate and produce a drier mixture.

Place the quince paste in an airtight vessel; refrigerate. Its color will deepen with time.

Nutrition Information

- Calories: 169 calories;

- Sodium: 3

- Total Carbohydrate: 44.1

- Cholesterol: 0

- Protein: 0.3

- Total Fat: 0.1

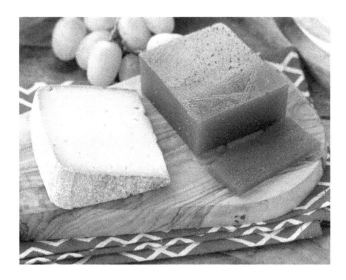

Remoulade Sauce A La New Orleans

Serving: 6

Ingredients

- 1 cup mayonnaise

- 1/4 cup chili sauce

- 2 tablespoons Creole mustard

- 2 tablespoons extra-virgin olive oil

- 1 tablespoon Louisiana-style hot sauce, or to taste

- 2 tablespoons fresh lemon juice

- 1 teaspoon Worcestershire sauce

- 4 medium scallions, chopped

- 2 tablespoons chopped fresh parsley

- 2 tablespoons chopped green olives

- 2 tablespoons minced celery

- 1 clove garlic, minced

- 1/2 teaspoon chili powder

- 1 teaspoon salt, or to taste

- 1/2 teaspoon ground black pepper

- 1 teaspoon capers, chopped (optional)

Direction

- Mix together the Worcestershire sauce, lemon juice, hot sauce, olive oil, mustard, chili sauce and mayonnaise.

- Mix in garlic, capers, celery, olives, parsley and scallions. Add pepper and salt and chili powder to season. Refrigerate with cover.

Nutrition Information

- Calories: 359 calories;

- Total Fat: 37.3

- Sodium: 943

- Total Carbohydrate: 6.7

- Cholesterol: 14

Roasted Eggplant And Tomato Towers

Serving: 4

Ingredients

- 6 large tomatoes, halved

- 1/2 cup olive oil, divided

- 2 cloves garlic, chopped

- 1 tablespoon dried oregano

- sea salt and ground black pepper to taste

- 1 large eggplant

- 1/2 teaspoon smoked paprika

- 1/2 cup plain yogurt

- 2 tablespoons honey

- 1/4 cup roasted almonds

Direction

- Start preheating the oven to 300°F (150°C).

- Put tomatoes with the cut side up on a cookie sheet. In a bowl, combine pepper, salt, oregano, garlic, and 1/4 cup of olive oil; put on the tomatoes.

- Put the tomatoes in the preheated oven and bake for 3-4 hours until slightly shrunken.

- In the last hour while the tomatoes are baking, cut eggplant into thin slices and use salt to drizzle, put aside for 30 minutes until some liquid starts to appear on the slices. Rinse the salt off the eggplant and move to a bowl. Put in the rest of the 1/4 cup olive oil and drizzle the eggplant slices with paprika. Use your hands to mix to so everything is coated.

- Put a layer of eggplant slices on a frying pan over medium heat and cook for 3-4 minutes until soft.

- Put the eggplant slices and tomato slices on serving dishes alternately, making 'towers.' Use honey and yogurt to sprinkle over each 'tower', put almonds on top.

Nutrition Information

- Calories: 425 calories;

- Cholesterol: 2

- Protein: 7.4

- Total Fat: 33

- Sodium: 119

- Total Carbohydrate: 31.1

Salmon Tartare

Serving: 2

Ingredients

- 1 (5 ounce) very fresh salmon fillet

- 1 teaspoon minced shallot

- 1 teaspoon minced fresh flat-leaf parsley

- 1 teaspoon minced fresh chives

- 1 teaspoon minced cornichon (small pickled cucumber)

- 1 teaspoon fresh lemon juice, or more to taste

- sea salt and freshly ground black pepper to taste

Direction

- Discard the salmon skin; take out the grey colored blood line so you can have shiny pink flesh only. Slice salmon into small dice and put in a bowl. Add in the pickle, lemon juice, parsley, chives, sea salt, pepper and shallot. Marinate for 5 minutes. Serve.

Nutrition Information

- Calories: 133 calories;

- Protein: 14.3

- Total Fat: 7.7

- Sodium: 227

- Total Carbohydrate: 0.6

- Cholesterol: 42

Salmon Tartare With Avocado Mousse

Serving: 4

Ingredients

- 1 1/2 pounds salmon fillets, cut into 1/4-inch cubes

- 1 tablespoon extra-virgin olive oil

- 1 tablespoon fresh lime juice

- 1 tablespoon fresh orange juice

- 1 teaspoon freshly ground pink peppercorns

- 1/2 teaspoon cream of balsamic (balsamic glaze)

- 2 tablespoons capers

- 2 tablespoons chopped fresh dill

- 12 chives

- Avocado Mousse:

- 2 firm-ripe California avocados, chilled

- 1/8 cup firm-ripe papaya flesh

- 1 tablespoon fresh lime juice

- 1 pinch salt

- 1/3 cup heavy cream, chilled

Direction

- In a bowl, put salmon, preferably wooden. In another bowl, mix balsamic cream, peppercorns, orange juice, lime juice, and olive oil. Add dill, capers, and dressing to the salmon. Gently toss but well.

- Decorate 3 chives on each plate.

- In a food processor, scoop avocado flesh. Put in salt, lime juice, and papaya; puree until smooth completely.

- Using an electric mixer, beat cream in a bowl until stiff peaks form. Gently fold avocado mixture in cream but thoroughly. It can be placed around tartare on a plate or served in a freestanding gravy boat.

Nutrition Information

- Calories: 582 calories;

- Cholesterol: 128

- Protein: 36.7

- Total Fat: 44

- Sodium: 283

- Total Carbohydrate: 11.5

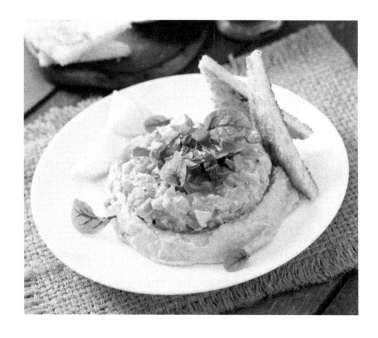

Sambousa

Serving: 10

Ingredients

- 1 pound lean ground beef

- 1/2 carrot, minced

- 1/2 onion, minced

- 1 clove garlic, minced

- 1 teaspoon tomato paste

- 1 green onion, chopped

- 1 pinch seasoning salt

- 1 green chile peppers, diced (optional)

- 1 (16 ounce) package egg roll wrappers, cut in half into rectangles

- 1 tablespoon all-purpose flour

- 1 tablespoon water

- 2 cups vegetable oil

Direction

- Brown the meat in a large skillet. Take the meat out from the skillet.

- Sauté green onion, carrot, garlic, and onion in the same skillet used to brown the meat. Put in the seasoning salt and tomato paste when the vegetables become tender. Add in the browned meat and stir.

- Blend the flour with water in a small bowl until forming a watery paste. In the front part of one of the strips, arrange 1 teaspoon full of the meat mixture. Beginning from the right front corner, fold over to the left. You've started the triangle shape. Carry on back and forth to shape into a triangle until there is no wrapper left. Use the water and the flour mixture to seal the wrappers. Repeat the process until there are no ingredients left.

- Taste with oil and fry the triangular packages until they become crisp. Then serve.

Nutrition Information

- Calories: 649 calories;

- Total Fat: 54.1

- Sodium: 318

- Total Carbohydrate: 28.1

- Cholesterol: 38

- Protein: 12.8

Samosas

Serving: 30

Ingredients

- 2 cups all-purpose flour

- 1/2 teaspoon salt

- 2 tablespoons butter

- 1/4 cup water

- 1 quart oil for deep frying

- 2 tablespoons butter

- 1 small onion, chopped

- 2 cloves garlic, chopped

- 2 green chile peppers, chopped

- 1 tablespoon fresh ginger root, chopped

- 1/2 teaspoon ground turmeric

- 1/2 teaspoon chili powder

- 3/4 pound ground lamb

- 1 teaspoon salt

- 2 teaspoons garam masala

- 1 1/2 tablespoons fresh lemon juice

Direction

- Combine butter, salt and flour in a medium bowl till mixture is similar to fine bread crumbs. Add in the water, putting additional up to about quarter cup if needed to create a smooth dough. Form into a round. Put on a slightly floured area and knead till dough is pliable and smooth for 10 minutes. Put back to bowl, place cover and reserve.

- In a big, deep skillet, heat the oil to 190 °C or 375 °F.

- In a medium saucepan, melt butter over medium high heat. Mix in ginger, green chili peppers, garlic and onion. Allow to cook for 5 minutes, or till onions turned golden brown. Mix in salt, ground lamb, chili powder and turmeric. Let cook for 10 minutes till lamb meat is equally brown. Mix in lemon juice and garam masala. Keep cooking for 5 minutes, then take off from heat.

- Distribute dough into 15 even pieces. Roll pieces forming rounds, then flatten create 4-inch circles. Halve every circle. Moistened edges and make cones out of semicircles. Stuff cones with even amount of lamb meat mixture. Moistened bottom and top edges of the cones, and pinch to secure.

- Into prepped oil, cautiously lower cones several at a time. Fry for 2 to 3 minutes till golden brown. Let drain on paper towels. Serve while warm.

Nutrition Information

- Calories: 105 calories;
- Protein: 2.9
- Total Fat: 7.3
- Sodium: 135

Savory Blue Cheese Cheesecake With Cherry Pear Compote And Cherry Balsamic Glaze

Serving: 24

Ingredients

- 1/2 cup butter

- 4 ounces freshly shredded Parmesan cheese

- 1 teaspoon minced fresh thyme leaves

- 1/2 teaspoon Kosher salt

- 1/2 teaspoon ground black pepper

- 1 1/4 cups all-purpose flour

- 1/4 cup chopped toasted pecans

- 1 tablespoon butter, melted

- 3 (8 ounce) packages cream cheese, softened

- 8 ounces blue cheese, crumbled

- 6 ounces freshly shredded Parmesan cheese

- 4 large eggs at room temperature

- 1/4 cup heavy cream at room temperature

- 1 teaspoon ground black pepper

- 2 tablespoons olive oil

- 2 large sweet onions, thinly sliced

- 2 pears - peeled, cored and chopped

- 1/2 cup dried cherries

- 2 tablespoons black cherry balsamic vinegar

- 1/2 cup brown sugar

- 1/4 teaspoon kosher salt

- 1 (8 ounce) package cream cheese

- 2 ounces freshly shredded Parmesan cheese

- 4 ounces blue cheese, crumbled

- 1/2 teaspoon ground black pepper

- 1/4 cup candied pecans

- 1 firm green pear, cored and thinly sliced

Direction

- In a big bowl, use an electric mixer to beat 1/2 tsp. black pepper, 1/2 tsp. salt, thyme, 4 ounces Parmesan cheese and 1/2 cup butter together until fluffy and light. Put in flour and mix on low speed until the mixture looks like big crumbles. Turn dough out and form into a log. Use plastic wrap to wrap the dough, then chill for an hour until cold.

- Set an oven to 175°C or 350°F. Slice the prepared dough into 1/4-inch thick pieces and put on a baking sheet.

- In the preheated oven, bake for 22 minutes until turn golden brown. Allow to crackers to cool on the sheets about 10 minutes before turning to a wire rack to cool thoroughly. Lower the heat of oven to 150°C or 300°F. Use parchment paper to line the bottom of a 10 inches springform pan, then coat the sides of pan and paper with butter.

- In a food processor, add 1 tbsp. melted butter, baked crackers and toasted pecans, then process until crumbled. Press into the bottom of prepared pan with the crumbs, then refrigerate in the fridge while making for the filling.

- In a big bowl, use an electric mixture to beat 6 ounces Parmesan cheese, 8 ounces blue cheese and three 8-ounce packages of cream cheese together until creamy and smooth. One at a time, put in eggs, allowing each egg to combine into the mixture before adding the next. Beat in the last egg together with 1 tsp. pepper and heavy cream. Transfer the mixture into the prepared pan.

- In the preheated oven, bake for 1 1/2 hours. Once the edges of cheesecake have nicely puffed and the surface is firm except for a small spot in the middle that will jiggle when the pan is shaken gently, it means the cheese cake is ready. Run around the edges of pan with the tip of a paring knife, then set the pan on a wire rack and let the cheesecake cool for an hour at room temperature before putting into the fridge to cool about 4 hours or overnight.

- In a skillet, heat olive oil on moderate heat. Stir in onion, then cook and stir for 5 minutes, until it turned translucent and has softened. Lower heat to moderately low and keep on cooking and stirring for 15-20 minutes longer, until the onion is dark brown and very tender. Put in 1/4 tsp. salt, brown sugar, balsamic vinegar, dried cherries and chopped pears, then cook and stir until pears are softened. Take the onion and fruit out of the skillet with a slotted spoon. Drain the juice back into skillet and use a fork to mash the fruit in a bowl. In the skillet, simmer the juice on moderate heat for 5 minutes, until thickened. Turn the glaze to a separate bowl.

- In a bowl, use an electric mixer to beat 1/2 tsp. black pepper, 2 ounces of Parmesan cheese, 4 ounces blue cheese and the leftover 8-ounce package of cream cheese together until smooth. Spread over the cooled cheesecake with the cheese mixture, then sprinkle over with candied pecans. Serve together with vinegar glaze, sliced pear and cheery pear compote on the side.

Nutrition Information

- Calories: 394 calories;
- Protein: 14.2
- Total Fat: 29.6
- Sodium: 651
- Total Carbohydrate: 19
- Cholesterol: 109

Savory Vegetarian Cream Puffs

Serving: 16

Ingredients

- Pastry Shells:

- 1 cup water

- 1/2 cup unsalted butter

- 2 tablespoons white sugar

- 1/2 teaspoon salt

- 1 cup all-purpose flour

- 4 eggs

- Filling:

- 10 1/2 ounces goat cheese

- 1 tablespoon dried dill weed

- salt to taste

Direction

Set oven to 220° C (425° F) and start preheating. Line a parchment paper or a silicone liner on a baking tray (or a baking stone).

In a saucepan on medium high heat, place salt, sugar, butter and water. Cook for 5 minutes, mixing occasionally, or till the mixture melts and dissolves. Decrease to medium heat. Add all of flour and cook for 15-30 seconds, mixing vigorously, or till a ball of dough is formed and it pulls away from sides of the pan.

Remove the dough to the bowl of a stand mixer fitted with a paddle attachment. Allow to cool for 5 minutes. Put in eggs, an egg at a time, whisking on medium-low speed after each addition, for 5 minutes, or till the batter is shiny and smooth.

Remove batter to a pastry bag fitted with a big round tip. Pipe into 2-in. mounds by squeezing close to the sheet and gradually pulling up.

Rise oven temperature to 230° C (450° F).

Put into the preheated and bake for 10 minutes until puffy. Decrease oven temperature to 175° C (350° F); keep baking for 13 to 15 minutes longer, or till shells are crispy and set.

In a stand mixer fitted with a whisk attachment, place salt, dill, and goat cheese. Mix for 2 to 3 minutes, or till filling is smooth and creamy. Pour into a pastry bag fitted with a small round tip, pipe filling into bottom of each shell until filled.

Nutrition Information

- Calories: 171 calories;
- Protein: 6.5
- Total Fat: 12.6
- Sodium: 197
- Total Carbohydrate: 8.2
- Cholesterol: 76

Scallop Ceviche

Serving: 4

Ingredients

- 1/2 pound fresh scallops, diced

- 2 clementines - peeled, segmented, and diced

- 1 Roma tomato, diced

- 1/2 small red onion

- 2 scallions, sliced

- 1/2 lemon, juiced

- 1/2 lime, juiced

- 1 clove garlic, minced

- 1 tablespoon chopped cilantro, or to taste (optional)

- 1/2 teaspoon olive oil

- sea salt to taste

Direction

- In a big bowl, mix together olive oil, cilantro, garlic, lime juice, lemon juice, scallions, red onion, tomato, clementines, and scallops. Put salt to season. Keep in the fridge for 2 hours until flavors blend, mixing from time to time.

Nutrition Information

- Calories: 109 calories;
- Sodium: 247
- Total Carbohydrate: 10
- Cholesterol: 34
- Protein: 15
- Total Fat: 1.3

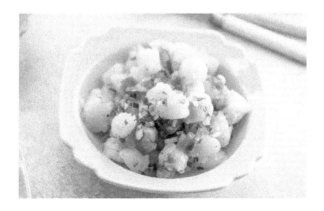

Scallop Ceviche De Gallo

Serving: 6

Ingredients

- 1 poblano chile pepper, halved lengthwise and seeded

- 1 serrano chile pepper, halved lengthwise and seeded

- 1 pound small bay scallops

- 1/2 cup fresh lime juice

- 4 tomatoes, diced, or more to taste

- 1 red onion, chopped

- 1/2 bunch fresh cilantro, chopped

- salt and ground black pepper to taste

Direction

Place the oven rack six inches from heat and preheat the broiler. Line the baking sheet with foil.

Put the Serrano chile and poblano peppers on the foil-lined baking sheet with the cut down.

Cook the peppers under broiler 5-8 minutes until the skin turns to black and blistered. Put the cooked peppers in a bowl then cover with plastic wrap tightly. Let it steam for 20 minutes. Peel the skins off then chop the flesh fine.

Boil a big pot of water. Add in the scallops and cook for about a minute. Drain the water out and transfer the scallops to a ceramic or glass bowl.

Pour the lime juice on top of the scallops. Add in the roasted peppers, onion, tomatoes, salt, cilantro and black pepper. Cover the mixture with plastic wrap then let it chill in the refrigerator for about 2 hours until scallops turn opaque and the flavors blend.

Put the ceviche into six martini glasses using a spoon to serve.

Nutrition Information

- Calories: 134 calories;
- Total Carbohydrate: 11.8
- Cholesterol: 46
- Protein: 20.5
- Total Fat: 1
- Sodium: 254

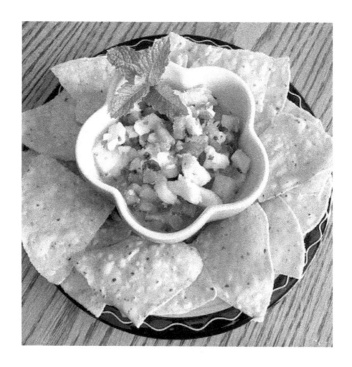

Shrimp Ramakis

Serving: 6

Ingredients

- 24 jumbo shrimp, peeled and deveined

- 1 1/2 cups bottled teriyaki sauce

- 1 pound bacon strips, cut in half

- 1 (8 ounce) can whole water chestnuts, drained

- 24 wooden toothpicks

Direction

- Toss teriyaki sauce and shrimp together in glass bowl. Use plastic wrap to cover and refrigerate to marinate for an hour.

- Place rack of oven to the center position and adjust the oven to heat.

- Take shrimp out of marinade; put each on 1/2 bacon strip with 1 water chestnut. Roll; secure using toothpick, then arrange, about half-inch away from each one, on broiler pan. Get rid of leftover marinade.

- Let ramakis broil about 5 minutes per side, or till bacon is cooked and shrimp turn pink (keep door of the oven slightly open and keep an eye). Transfer onto paper towels to drain; serve right away.

Nutrition Information

- Calories: 366 calories;

- Total Fat: 12.9

- Sodium: 3547

- Total Carbohydrate: 17.4

- Cholesterol: 240

- Protein: 42.3

Shrimp And Tortellini Skewers

Serving: 12

Ingredients

- 36 fresh cheese tortellini

- 1 tablespoon olive oil

- 1 tablespoon minced garlic

- 24 large cooked shrimp

- 12 skewers

- 12 cherry tomatoes

- Dip:

- 1 (16 ounce) container sour cream

- 1 (1 ounce) package dry ranch dressing mix (such as Hidden Valley Ranch®)

Direction

- Boil a big pot of lightly salted water; add tortellini. Cook for 2-3 minutes until al dente; drain.

- On medium heat, heat olive oil in a pan; add garlic. Cook and stir for 1-2 minutes until tender and aromatic; add shrimp. Cook for 2-3 minutes until the shrimp is heated through. Toss tortellini in the shrimp mixture. Take off heat and let it cool until it can be handled easily.

- In a skewer, lace tortellini and shrimp alternately with the tomato at the end. Repeat with the leftover ingredients.

- In a bowl, combine ranch dressing mix and sour cream. Serve skewers with the mixture.

Nutrition Information

- Calories: 374 calories;

- Total Fat: 16.6

- Sodium: 522

- Total Carbohydrate: 42.7

- Cholesterol: 73

- Protein: 15

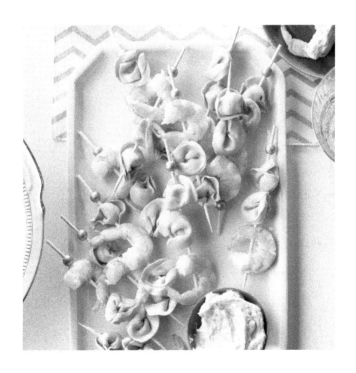

Shrimp De Jonghe I

Serving: 4

Ingredients

- 1 1/2 pounds shrimp, peeled and deveined

- 2 cups dry white wine

- 1 cup butter, melted

- 2 cloves garlic, minced

- 1 pinch ground cayenne pepper

- 1/2 teaspoon paprika

- 1 cup chopped fresh parsley

- 2 cups fresh bread crumbs

Direction

- Preheat an oven to 175°C (350°F). Lightly spread over a casserole dish of 11x 7 inches with cooking spray.

- Put shrimp in the casserole plate uniformly. Drizzle wine over the shrimp.

- Stir bread crumbs, parsley, paprika, cayenne pepper, garlic and butter. Top the shrimp with sprinkle of bread crumb mixture. If required, refrigerate instantly.

- Bake for 20 minutes in a preheated oven, until the topping is golden brown and shrimp is firm. Serve right away.

Nutrition Information

- Calories: 864 calories;

- Cholesterol: 381

- Protein: 36.2

- Total Fat: 50.5

- Sodium: 1035

- Total Carbohydrate: 43.9

Simply Marinated Mushrooms

Serving: 6

Ingredients

- 1 cup water

- 1 1/2 pounds fresh mushrooms, stems removed

- 1/4 cup olive oil

- 1 teaspoon dried thyme

- 1 teaspoon salt

- 3 tablespoons fresh lemon juice

- 3 teaspoons minced garlic

- 1/2 teaspoon ground black pepper

- 3 tablespoons dried parsley

- 1/8 teaspoon onion powder

Direction

- In a large pot, boil water. Stir in mushrooms and simmer for about 10 minutes. Take away from heat and drain.

- In a large bowl, whisk the thyme, olive oil, lemon juice, salt, pepper, garlic, onion powder and parsley together. Add mushrooms and toss to coat. Refrigerate to marinade overnight, and rewarm when serving.

Nutrition Information

- Calories: 115 calories;

- Total Fat: 9.5

- Sodium: 393

- Total Carbohydrate: 7.2

- Cholesterol: 0

- Protein: 2.5

Smoked Salmon Mousse

Serving: 16

Ingredients

- 4 ounces smoked salmon

- 2 tablespoons heavy cream

- 1 (8 ounce) package cream cheese, softened

- 1/2 lemon, juiced

- 1/2 teaspoon dried dill weed to taste

- salt and pepper to taste

- 1 ounce salmon roe

Direction

- In a food processor or blender, put the smoked salmon and process until smooth.

- Add in cream cheese, dried dill weed, pepper, salt, heavy cream and half of a lemon's juice.

- Continue processing until consistency desired is achieved. Transfer dip into a serving bowl and add salmon roe as garnish.

Nutrition Information

- Calories: 67 calories;

- Total Carbohydrate: 0.8

- Cholesterol: 26

- Protein: 2.8

- Total Fat: 6

- Sodium: 99

Spanakopita II

Ingredients

- 1/2 cup vegetable oil

- 2 large onions, chopped

- 2 (10 ounce) packages frozen chopped spinach - thawed, drained and squeezed dry

- 2 tablespoons chopped fresh dill

- 2 tablespoons all-purpose flour

- 2 (4 ounce) packages feta cheese, crumbled

- 4 eggs, lightly beaten

- salt and pepper to taste

- 1 1/2 (16 ounce) packages phyllo dough

- 3/4 pound butter, melted

Direction

- Preheat the oven to 175°C or 350°Fahrenheit.

- On medium heat, heat vegetable oil in a big pot. Cook and stir onions slowly until soft. Stir in flour, dill and spinach. Cook for about 10 minutes until nearly all the moisture is absorbed. Take off from the heat; mix in pepper, salt, eggs and feta cheese.

- Separate one phyllo sheet from the stack and brush evenly with a thin coat of butter. Put another phyllo sheet on top of the butter then press the 2 phyllo sheets together. Make 3-in wide long strips from the layered phyllo dough. Keep the rest of the phyllo sheets covered in plastic wrap to avoid drying out.

- On a work surface, place one phyllo strip at a time with one of the slender ends near you. Put a heaping tablespoonful of filling an inch from the end nearest to you. Fold the lower right corner over the filling then to the left corner to make a triangle. Fold it up joining the point at the lower left up to lay along the left corner. Turn the bottom left edge to touch the right corner. Continue to fold the triangle over in this way until you reach the phyllo's end.

- Repeat with the rest of the phyllo dough and filling. Arrange the filled phyllo dough triangles on a big baking sheet then slather with the rest of the butter. You can freeze the pastries at this point.

- Bake the phyllo in the preheated oven for 45 minutes to an hour until golden brown.

Nutrition Information

- Calories: 246 calories;

- Sodium: 313

- Total Carbohydrate: 15.9

- Cholesterol: 62

- Protein: 5

- Total Fat: 18.4

Spiced Bacon Twists

Serving: 8

Ingredients

- 1 cup packed light brown sugar

- 2 tablespoons dry mustard powder

- 1/2 teaspoon ground cinnamon

- 1/2 teaspoon ground nutmeg

- 1/4 teaspoon cayenne pepper

- 1 pound sliced bacon

Direction

- Start preheating the oven to 350°F (175°C). Use an aluminum foil to line a cookie sheet and put a wire rack over the foil. Catch the grease with a sided cookie sheet.

- Combine cayenne pepper, nutmeg, cinnamon, mustard powder, and brown sugar in a small bowl. Dip to coat the bacon strips in the mixture. Twist each strips several times and put on the prepared baking rack.

- Put in the preheated oven and bake for 30 minutes until the bacon strips are crunchy enough to maintain its shape and turn brown.

Nutrition Information

- Calories: 219 calories;

- Total Fat: 8.7

- Sodium: 438

- Total Carbohydrate: 28

- Cholesterol: 20

- Protein: 7.6

Spicy Potato Noodles (Bataka Sev)

Serving: 8

Ingredients

- For the Green Chile Paste:

- 1/4 cup chopped fresh green chile peppers

- 1 tablespoon coarsely chopped garlic

- 2 tablespoons fresh ginger, peeled and coarsely chopped

- 1 teaspoon salt

- 1/8 teaspoon ground turmeric

- 2 teaspoons vegetable oil

- For the Noodles:

- 1 pound potatoes, peeled

- 3 cups water

- 3 1/2 cups chickpea flour

- 2 1/2 teaspoons salt

- 1 teaspoon ground turmeric

- 2 tablespoons mustard oil

- vegetable oil for deep frying

Direction

- In a mortar and pestle or food processor, mix 2 teaspoons of vegetable oil, 1/8 teaspoon of turmeric, 1 teaspoon salt, ginger, garlic and chiles. Then process to form a fine paste. (If you need more liquid, pour in 1 tablespoon water). Put aside.

- Put potatoes in a saucepan along with water and then heat to a boil on high heat. Decrease the heat to low and cover the pan. Cook potatoes for about 15 minutes until soft and easily pricked with a fork. Save the cooking water.

- Mash potatoes while still warm and add some of the cooking water to have a smooth consistency. Stir in mustard oil, 1 teaspoon turmeric, 2 1/2 teaspoons salt, chickpea flour and 1 tablespoon green chile paste. Pour in enough of the reserved potato-cooking water as needed to form a soft dough. Check the seasoning and heat lever of the dough (dough should taste raw but should be spicy and salty. Flavors will mellow slightly while cooking). If desired, add more chile paste and salt.

- Over medium-high heat, heat cooking oil in a deep pan. Press noodles into the oil with a potato ricer (or use sev machine, if lucky to have it). Fry for about 2 minutes until crisp and golden brown. Place noodles onto a bowl lined with paper towel with the help of a skimmer or slotted spoon. Repeat this until all of the noodles are fried. Keep in an airtight container for a maximum of 2 weeks.

Nutrition Information

- Calories: 336 calories;
- Total Fat: 18.4
- Sodium: 1024
- Total Carbohydrate: 35.2
- Cholesterol: 0
- Protein: 9.4

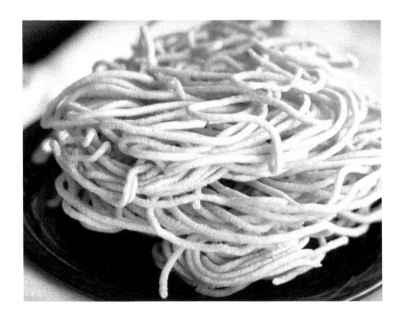

Spicy Sweet Stovetop Popcorn

Serving: 4

Ingredients

- 2 tablespoons coconut oil

- 3 tablespoons agave nectar

- 2 tablespoons dried chipotle chili pepper

- 1/2 cup unpopped popcorn

Direction

- In a large saucepan or soup pot over medium-high heat, heat chipotle powder, agave nectar and coconut oil.

- Once the blend begins to have small bubbles, pour in the popcorn and mix it to cover the kernels with a fork. Cover the pan with a lid.

- When the corn begins popping, constantly shake the pan until the popping quits. Expel from heat, and pour popped corn in a big bowl.

Nutrition Information

- Calories: 202 calories;

- Total Fat: 8.3

- Sodium: 2

- Total Carbohydrate: 31.3

- Cholesterol: 0

- Protein: 3.2

THANK YOU

Thank you for choosing *Fresh and Healthy Salads and Appetizers* for improving your cooking skills! I hope you enjoyed making the recipes as much as tasting them! If you're interested in learning new recipes and new meals to cook, go and check out the other books of the series.

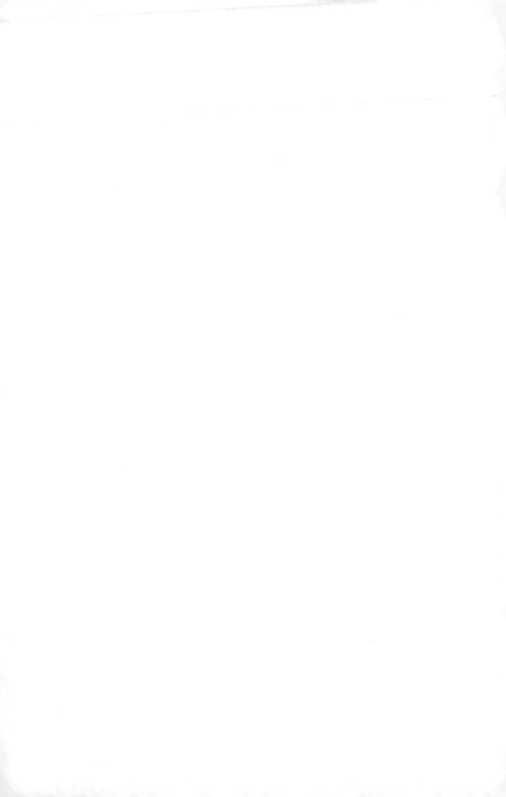

Lightning Source UK Ltd.
Milton Keynes UK
UKHW022001020421
381458UK00003B/140

9 781802 230871